The

-- Complete --

Crohnie

Handbook

A
Comprehensive
Guide for the
Crohn's Disease Patient

ROBERT R. PILKINGTON

- The Complete Crohnie Handbook -

A Comprehensive Guide for the
Crohn's Disease Patient

ISBN: 0-9718871-0-1

SAN 2 5 5 – 1 7 7 2

Library of Congress Control Number:

2002102863

Crohnie

is a Registered Trademark
of Robert Pilkington

Professional Medical Treatment and Disclaimer

The material in this Handbook is provided for your information and education only. You should never treat yourself for a medical condition or decide that you do not need medical treatment based on the information contained in this Handbook. In other words, the information available throughout this Handbook should not be interpreted as medical or professional advice. All medical information contained in this Handbook or any other source needs to be reviewed carefully with your own doctor before you act upon it in any way. If you are sick, you must to go to the doctor. No exceptions!

With respect to the information contained in this Handbook, the Author, the editing staff and any other parties involved in the creation, production or delivery of this Handbook are not liable for any direct, incidental, consequential, indirect, or punitive damages arising out of your access to, or use of this Handbook. The Author is providing this Handbook and its contents on an "as is" basis and makes no representation or warranty of any kind with respect to this Handbook or its contents. The Author disclaims all such representations and warranties.

Likewise, the Author disclaims any legal liability or responsibility for the accuracy, completeness, or usefulness of any information, procedure, method, apparatus, product, or process identified in this Handbook. The Author assumes no responsibility for loss or damages resulting from the use of information contained in this Handbook.

Any reference made in this Handbook to any specific commercial product, process, or service by trade name, trademark, manufacturer, or otherwise does not indicate or imply that the Author endorses, recommends, or favors the items mentioned.

Editor in Chief
Denise L. Pilkington

Contributing Editors:

Robert Pilkington

Dr. Gerald Wolfley

Dr. Robert Leon

Jason Schultz

Katherine Murphy

Marc Carleno

Leo Farrier

This book is dedicated to June and Leo Farrier

Mom and Dad

"… and I think to myself, what a wonderful world."

Louis Armstrong

Acknowledgments

Gracious acknowledgments and thanks are made to Dr. Gerald Wolfley, Dr. William Marsh and Dr. Robert Leon. After a physician who was not properly educated about Crohn's disease misdiagnosed my illness and performed a surgical procedure that nearly killed me, these men came to my rescue and were able to diagnose my Crohn's and properly treat it, thus saving my life. Without these three outstanding physicians along with the support of their fine staff members I would not be here today.

Special thanks are given to Dr. Wolfley who has zero tolerance when I miss or cancel an appointment and who never seems to forget what my triglyceride levels are.

Sadly, Dr. Wolfley passed away on September 3, 2002, after a long illness. He was respected and loved by all of his patients and was a well respected physician in the community. Dr. Wolfley will be missed by everyone who had the pleasure to know this fine physician and caring man.

Thanks are also given to those who edited this Handbook helping to make its publication a reality.

Robert R. Pilkington was diagnosed with Crohn's disease on May 26, 1990. He was 29 years old. His first recorded day of sickness was August 8, 1988. Between these dates, Robert had three major surgical procedures performed and nearly lost his life because of an incorrect diagnosis and an improperly performed surgical procedure. Robert suffered debilitating and life-long damage to his body because of one surgical mistake. Because of the misdiagnosis, Robert's colon eventually ruptured and the damage was so severe that 2/3 of the colon was removed.

Robert also suffers many other health-related problems that are a direct result of Crohn's disease. At the writing of this Handbook, Robert has been a Crohnie for over 12 years.

Since he copes with many of the same symptoms, sicknesses, problems, public embarrassments and fears that most of you do, he understands what you have to live with, everyday, with no real end in sight. He also requires the same support, guidance and understanding that each of you does. Through this Handbook he hopes to provide some of that support, guidance and understanding about day to day life and what to do if you do have a relapse.

As a result of his constant and on-going daily battle with Crohn's disease, Robert has experienced almost all of the local and systemic side effects of the disease. He has also taken most of the medications available to Crohn's patients and has experienced most of the side effects of each.

Because of his Crohn's disease, Robert's weight dropped from 298 pounds on April 10, 1990 to 164 pounds on Christmas Day of that same year. In less than 7 months he went from playing semi-professional football with the Maricopa County Sheriff's Department to being almost bed ridden. His low point came when he had become so weak that he was unable to mow his lawn and had to ask his father to do it for him.

Robert has been fortunate because through diet and exercise, he found a way to control his Crohn's and again weighs over 200 pounds. Robert exercises and lifts weights regularly and has developed a diet and supplement routine that contains high protein, complex carbohydrates, balanced fiber, essential fatty acids, supplements and amino acids; a diet that he follows every day with very little changes in his day to day routine. He developed his diet through years of trial and error and finding out what his body would and would not tolerate.

Robert was able to maintain his disease from December 1991 until October 2001 at which time he knew he was having a relapse. He was able to get to his doctor before his symptoms got too severe but even with that, he was sick for three months. As he has learned, the biggest challenge facing a Crohnie is knowing the difference between just being sick and actually having a relapse of the disease. By the way a Crohnie feels most days he knows that sometimes it's hard to tell the difference.

Robert holds a Bachelor of Science degree in Business Administration from the University of Phoenix and has earned a Certification in Procurement from UCLA. He is a member of the National Contract

Management Association and has won several awards in Training, Negotiation, Management and Legal Writing & Editing.

Robert has trained the Procurement and Sales staff of several major corporations in the Phoenix area, has been a certified auditor for two Fortune 500 companies and was a certified ISO auditor for a division of one of the largest automobile manufacturers in the world.

Robert is the former Managing Director for The Automotive-Sales Training Group in Scottsdale, Arizona. The Automotive-Sales Training Group training modules that Robert personally developed specialize in training automobile Sales Professionals by promoting ethical behavior, honesty, hands on experience and classroom instruction. He currently owns *Justice for Judgments*, a Casa Grande, Arizona company dedicated to recovering debts for people who have been awarded monetary judgments in court, and for whatever reason, have been unable to collect payment from the judgment debtor.

Robert is not a doctor nor is he a research professional. The information contained in this handbook is a result of his personal experiences, research and what has worked for him in the treatment and maintenance of the disease.

This Crohnie Handbook came into being at the request of several of my friends and family members as I have done a tremendous amount of research on Crohn's disease and they all felt that I had acquired some valuable information about the disease and how to deal with it. Through trial and error, I have learned many different ways to keep my Crohn's under control and because I understand that there is no one exact standard about Crohn's disease treatment, the main purpose of this Handbook is to share a multitude of information with you and provide you with a reference tool that you can use to help you further understand your Crohn's. I also hope to provide some thoughts on how to keep your Crohn's under control with the realization that some suggestions may work and some may not. Your success is going to depend on your individual case, symptoms, environment and condition.

I will use laymen's terms and easy to understand English but I will have to use some technical and medical terms to tie it all together. Any technical or medical term that needs clarification will be defined. Also included are some reference information, medication information, medication side effects, vitamins and supplements, nutritional information, some support organizations and some helpful websites.

Many books have been written about Crohn's disease by those who have only studied or treated it and most books are written by more than one person. But for those of us who live with it from day to day, every day of our entire lives, we know what it is like to be sick by ourselves with no end in sight. This Handbook has been written from that perspective.

Even when I have my Crohn's somewhat under control, I too endure the long sleepless nights, the pain, agony, suffering, loneliness, public embarrassment, and the fear that those who don't have this disease won't really understand what we are going through. It is hard to explain that we are sick when we appear to be perfectly healthy.

As I have found in my research of Crohn's disease and other chronic illnesses, most people with Crohn's don't complain too much about being sick, but the sick feeling never goes away. I have also discovered that there are many support groups with many people who suffer greatly from Crohn's and you should make every attempt to become involved with some of these groups. The only way to know more about your disease is to know more about your disease.

Hopefully, this Handbook will assist you to understand Crohn's disease a little better and help you to cope with and overcome that never-ending sick feeling.

Contents

Introduction

If you have Crohn's disease, don't feel alone. Over 500,000 Americans have the disease, accounting for approximately 75,000 hospitalizations per year. The cost of the disease in 1990, the year I was diagnosed, was about $1.2 billion. Today, the cost of lost workdays alone by Crohn's patients is estimated at a half-billion dollars a year. It is believed that there may be up to 2,000,000 Americans with Crohn's disease or ulcerative colitis.

Males and females appear to be affected equally and while Crohn's afflicts people of all ages it is primarily a disease of the young with most cases being diagnosed before age 30. About 50% of Crohn's patients are free of symptoms at any given time but the vast majority suffers at least one relapse in any 5 year period. While drug treatment is effective for about 70 - 80% of patients, surgery becomes necessary in the remaining 20 - 30%.

In her 1969 book *On Death and Dying*, Dr. Elisabeth Kubler-Ross proposed and defined the 5 stages of death and dying. These stages are often called "the five stages of grief" and are:

Denial
Anger
Depression
Bargaining
Acceptance

Since her book was published, Dr. Kubler-Ross' work has been applied not only to death, dying and grief, but also to the onset of a chronic illness. There is no time limit set for each stage as every person progresses toward the final stage of Acceptance at their own pace. Some people may experience more than one stage at a time or in an alternate order. Accordingly, some critics have argued that these steps may be too rigid thus are not applicable to the Acceptance process. Yet many people around the world have found her work to be very much a part of their lives.

The first stage in acceptance of a chronic illness like Crohn's disease is *Denial.* You may convince yourself that the lab reports or your doctor are wrong, but when someone is diagnosed with Crohn's neither the lab reports nor the doctor are usually wrong. With the often sudden onset of Crohn's, it can be easy to believe that symptoms are food poisoning, the flu, or due to stress, and the symptoms will eventually go away. You might even refuse to take medication or alter your diet. Regardless of what you do, Crohn's disease is real and it is with you to stay.

The second stage is *Anger.* Your anger may be directed at your doctor, your family or your friends. Your anger may be directed at the illness itself or it may even be directed at the rest of the world for going on about its business as if nothing has happened to you. One thing that is almost guaranteed is that if you spend too much time at this stage, it will leave you feeling resentful and bitter of healthy people. Friends and family may even turn away from you if you get stuck in this stage too long.

Bargaining is the third stage. You may rationalize with yourself that eating unhealthily or not taking your meds is ok by using the excuse that, "One day of missing my meds won't hurt". My personal favorite excuse is

"I'll schedule my colonoscopy when I'm not so busy"; which is never ... so you get my point. Unfortunately your Crohn's isn't going away for the weekend or taking a break for the holidays and your Crohn's doesn't care that a colonoscopy is something you would rather avoid because you are "just too busy".

The fourth stage, one that is familiar to anyone diagnosed with a chronic illness, is *Depression*. You may feel sorry for yourself and lose hope of ever achieving remission. Don't feel alone as this is a common feeling. My own depression lasted almost 7 years before I was able to overcome it, and during that time, I did have thoughts of taking my life. It is important to recognize that medical help is necessary if depression becomes all consuming or results in suicidal thoughts. Adjusting to a chronic illness is a difficult and stressful process. Seeking out help, support, solace and information about how to deal with it is the best way to ensure a more healthy life.

The fifth and final stage is *Acceptance*. As said before, your Crohn's is not going to go away, and becoming educated about the disease is the way to lead a healthier life. By taking the time to become better educated about this disease, you are headed in the right direction.

Dr. Kubler-Ross' 5 stages provide a guideline in the lonely and perilous journey to accepting Crohn's as a part of your life. That is not to say that Crohn's should rule your life or that the search for a cause and cure should stop, but you must make and keep regular doctors appointments and take your meds as required. Doctor visits and meds are going to be a part of your life, but hopefully a very small part of it. You should try to live a life that is filled with success, happiness, and many incredible experiences ... despite the illness you have.

I hope that when you are done reading this Handbook you will have been able to gain some understanding about the disease that is a part of your life and you will refer to this Handbook often. I have not been able to find a *complete and thorough* publication on Crohn's disease that has been written by someone who has Crohn's disease and understands the disease and how it affects the body and mind. What I have found, is the "3 page information sheets" that don't give all the information or explain next to nothing, a few other pamphlets that have little if any useful information on them, and technical or medical books that confused me more than helped me. I needed to have information about my disease and be able to understand what I was dealing with in a language and written in terminology that meant something to me when I read it.

Those reasons along with being pushed along by friends and family is why I decided to write this Handbook. I wanted others to have the benefit of the many hours I spent learning about this disease, the affect that it has on our day-to-day life as well as treatments, maintenance and the long-term effects ... written in a format that is not intimidating and could be easily understood.

Chapter 1

The Digestive System

The digestive system is a complex series of hollow organs that are responsible for converting the food that is eaten into the nutrients that are required to fuel the body's metabolism. The term *gastrointestinal tract* refers to the entire digestive system. The simplest explanation is that the digestive system it is a tube running from mouth to anus.

Inside the digestive system is a lining called the mucosa and in the mouth, stomach, and small intestine, the mucosa contains tiny glands that produce juices to help breakdown food. There are also two solid digestive organs, the liver and the pancreas, which produce juices that reach the intestine through small tubes. Additionally, parts of other organ systems play a major role in the digestive system.

This following section of this Chapter is a guide to describe the various components of the digestive system and how each works.

The Digestive Process

When we eat any food it is not in a form that the body can use as nourishment. The food and drink that we consume must be changed into smaller molecules of nutrients before they can be absorbed into the blood and carried to cells throughout the body. The digestive system serves as a sort of an assembly line, or more distinctly, a disassembly line. Its main goal is to break

21

down macromolecules which are proteins, fats and starch into smaller molecules, known as amino acids, fatty acids and glucose. The smaller molecules are then absorbed across the wall of the tube, and into the circulatory system for dissemination throughout your body. This process is known as digestion.

Digestion is accomplished through a combination of mechanical and enzymatic processes. For the body to digest food and drink, the digestive system requires considerable assistance from accessory digestive organs such as the salivary glands, liver and pancreas, which dump their secretions into the system. Without pancreatic enzymes you would starve to death in a very short time.

The Digestive System's Regulators

A fascinating feature of the digestive system is that it contains its own regulators. The major hormones that control the functions of the digestive system are produced and released by cells in the mucosa of the stomach and small intestine. These hormones are released into the blood of the digestive tract, travel back to the heart and through the arteries, and return to the digestive system, where they stimulate digestive juices and cause organ movement. The hormones that control digestion are gastrin, secretin, and cholecystokinin (CCK).

Gastrin causes the stomach to produce an acid for dissolving and digesting some foods. It is also necessary for the normal growth of the lining of the stomach, small intestine, and colon.

Secretin causes the pancreas to send out a digestive juice that is rich in bicarbonate. It stimulates the stomach to produce pepsin, an enzyme that digests protein, and it also stimulates the liver to produce bile.

CCK causes the pancreas to grow and to produce the enzymes of pancreatic juice and it causes the gallbladder to empty.

The Digestive System's Nerves

Two types of nerves help to control the action of the digestive system. Extrinsic, or outside nerves, come to the digestive organs from the unconscious part of the brain or from the spinal cord. They release a chemical called acetylcholine and another called adrenaline. Acetylcholine causes the muscle of the digestive organs to squeeze with more force and increase the push of food and juice through the digestive system. Acetylcholine also causes the stomach and pancreas to produce more digestive juice. Adrenaline relaxes the muscle of the stomach and intestine and decreases the flow of blood to these organs.

Even more important are the intrinsic or inside nerves. These nerves make up a very dense network embedded in the walls of the esophagus, stomach, small intestine, and colon. The intrinsic nerves are triggered to act when the walls of the hollow organs are stretched by food. These nerves cause the release of many different substances that speed up or delay the movement of food and the production of juices by the digestive organs.

Proper function of the digestive system requires healthy regulators and nerves. These regulators and nerves must facilitate communication among different sections of the digestive system and between the digestive system and the brain. Control of digestive function is achieved through a combination of electrical and hormonal messages which originate either within the digestive system's own nervous and endocrine systems or from the central nervous system and its endocrine organs, such as the adrenal gland.

The Production of Digestive Juices

The glands that act first in producing digestive juices are in the mouth. They are called the salivary glands. Saliva produced by these glands contains an enzyme that begins to digest the starch from food into smaller molecules. These juices also act as a lubricant to help move the food through the digestive system.

The next set of digestive glands is in the stomach lining. They produce stomach acid and an enzyme that digests protein. One of the greatest unsolved mysteries of the human body is why the acid juice of the stomach does not dissolve the tissue of the stomach itself. In most people, the stomach mucosa is able to resist the juice, although food and other tissues of the body cannot.

When the stomach empties the food and its juice into the small intestine the digestive juices of two other organs mix with the food to continue the process of digestion.

One of these organs is the pancreas. The pancreas produces a juice that contains a wide array of enzymes to break down the carbohydrates, fat, and protein in our food. Other enzymes that are active in the process come from glands in the wall of the intestine.

The other organ, the liver, produces its own digestive juice. It is called bile and is stored between meals in the gallbladder. At mealtime, bile is squeezed out of the gallbladder into the bile ducts to reach the intestine and mix with the fat in our food. The bile acids dissolve the fat into the watery contents of the intestine, much like detergents dissolve grease from a greasy pan. After the fat is dissolved, enzymes from the pancreas and the lining of the intestine digest it.

Peristalsis

Peristalsis is a distinctive pattern of smooth muscle contractions that propels foodstuffs distally through the esophagus and intestines by contraction above and relaxation below the segment being stimulated.

Absorption and Transport of Nutrients

Digested molecules of food, as well as water and minerals from the diet, are absorbed from the cavity of the upper small intestine. The absorbed materials cross the mucosa into the blood, and are carried off in the bloodstream to other parts of the body for storage or further chemical change.

The five following subtitles define how the digestive system digests the different types of food and liquid that we eat and drink.

Carbohydrates

An average American adult eats about half a pound of carbohydrate each day. Some of our most common foods, like bread, potatoes, pastries, candy, rice, spaghetti, fruits and vegetables, contain mostly carbohydrates. Many of these foods also contain starch which can be digested and many of these foods also contain fiber. The body cannot digest fiber.

The digestible carbohydrates are broken into simpler molecules by enzymes in the saliva, in juice produced by the pancreas, and in the lining of the small intestine. Starch is digested in two steps: First, an enzyme in the saliva and pancreatic juice breaks the starch into molecules called maltose; then an enzyme in the lining of the small intestine splits the maltose into glucose molecules that can be absorbed into the blood. Glucose is carried through the bloodstream to the liver, where it is stored or used to provide energy for the work of the body.

Table sugar is another carbohydrate that must be digested to be useful. An enzyme in the lining of the small intestine digests table sugar into glucose and fructose, each of which can be absorbed from the intestinal cavity into the blood. Milk contains yet another type of sugar, lactose, which is changed into absorbable molecules by an enzyme called lactase, also found in the intestinal lining. Many people with Crohn's disease are lactose intolerant, meaning they cannot properly digest or process lactose.

Proteins

Foods such as meat, eggs, and beans consist of giant molecules of protein that must be digested by enzymes before they can be used to build and repair body tissues. An enzyme in the juice of the stomach starts the digestion of swallowed protein. Further digestion of the protein is completed in the small intestine. Here, several enzymes from the pancreatic juice and the lining of the intestine carry out the breakdown of huge protein molecules into small molecules called amino acids. These small molecules can be absorbed from the hollow of the small intestine into the blood and then be carried to all parts of the body to build the walls and other parts of cells.

Fats

Fat molecules are a rich source of energy for the body. The first step in digestion of fat is to dissolve it into the watery content of the intestinal cavity. The bile acids produced by the liver act as natural detergents to dissolve fat in water and allow the enzymes to break the large fat molecules into smaller molecules, some of which are fatty acids and cholesterol. The bile acids combine with the fatty acids and cholesterol and help these molecules to move into the cells of the mucosa. In these cells, the small molecules are formed back into large molecules, most of which pass into vessels, called lymphatic, near the intestine. These small vessels carry the reformed fat to the veins of the chest, and the blood carries the fat to storage depots in different parts of the body.

Vitamins

Another vital part of our food that is absorbed from the small intestine is the class of chemicals known as vitamins. There are two different types of vitamins, classified by the fluid in which they can be dissolved: water-soluble vitamins, which are all the B vitamins and vitamin C; and fat-soluble vitamins, which are vitamins A, D, and K. These Vitamins are all discussed later in the Handbook.

Water and Salt

Most of the material absorbed from the cavity of the small intestine is water, in which salt is dissolved. The salt and water come from the food and liquid we swallow and the juices secreted by the many digestive glands. In a healthy adult, more than a gallon of water containing over an ounce of salt is absorbed from the intestine every 24 hours.

The Anatomy of the Digestive System

The Mouth

The first part of the digestive system is the mouth. The purpose of the mouth is to break down food by chewing. Saliva assists in the breakdown process and is added as a lubricant.

The Esophagus

When you eat and swallow your food, it enters the next part of the digestive system, which is called the esophagus. The esophagus is the organ into which the swallowed food is pushed. It connects the throat above with the stomach below. From the esophagus, the food then moves relatively quickly to the stomach where it is initially digested. The stomach reduces the food to a liquid form. As food is liquefied in the stomach it passes through the pyloric canal into the small intestine.

At the intersection or junction of the esophagus and stomach, there is a ring like valve, called the pyloric sphincter, closing the passage between the two organs. As the food approaches the closed ring, the surrounding muscles relax and allow the food to pass.

The Stomach

The stomach is an expanded section of the digestive tube between the esophagus and small intestine. The right side of the stomach is called the greater curvature and the left the lesser curvature. The most distal and narrow section of the stomach is termed the pylorus.

The wall of the stomach is structurally similar to other parts of the digestive tube except the stomach has an extra oblique layer of smooth muscle inside the circular layer. This aids in performance of complex grinding motions. When the stomach is empty, it is contracted and its mucosa and submucosa are thrown up into distinct folds called rugae. When filled with food, the rugae are ironed out and flat.

The stomach has four major types of secretory epithelial cells that cover the surface of the stomach and extend down into gastric pits and glands of the stomach. The first are the Mucous cells which secrete alkaline mucus that protects the epithelium against shear stress and acid. The second are the Parietal cells. These cells secrete hydrochloric acid. The third cells are Chief cells, which secrete a proteolytic enzyme known as pepsin. And fourth are the G cells, which secrete the hormone gastrin.

There are differences in the distribution of these cell types among regions of the stomach. For example, parietal cells are abundant in the glands of the body, but virtually absent in pyloric glands. The other cell types are farther down in the pits.

The final task of the stomach is to empty its contents slowly into the small intestine. The pyloric sphincter controls movement of food from the stomach to the small intestine.

The Small Intestine

Several factors affect emptying of the stomach, including the nature of the food and the degree of muscle action required by the stomach and the small intestine. As the food is digested in the small intestine and dissolved into the juices from the pancreas, liver, and intestine, the contents of the intestine are mixed and pushed forward to allow further digestion.

The main function of the small intestine is to absorb nutrients from the food particles that are passed to it from the stomach. The food is further digested in the small intestine with the assistance of secretions from the liver, gall bladder and pancreas.

The small intestine is about 20 feet long and is also referred to as small bowel. The small intestine is the longest section of the digestive tube and consists of three segments forming a passage from the stomach to the large intestine.

The three parts of the small intestine are the duodenum, which is the part nearest the stomach; the jejunum, which is the middle of the small intestines; and the ileum, which connects the small intestine to the large intestine. The ileum, known as the terminal ileum, is a frequent site of involvement of the digestive system in Crohn's disease.

A bulk of the small intestine is suspended from the body wall by an extension of the peritoneum called the mesentery and blood vessels to and from the intestine lie between the two sheets of the mesentery. Lymphatic vessels are also present.

It is within the small intestine that the final stages of digestion occur using enzymes and transforming the food particles into small molecules capable of being absorbed. The small intestine is also the sole site in the digestive tube for absorption of amino acids and sugars and carbohydrates, known as monosaccharides. Most lipids are also absorbed in this organ. All of this absorption and much of the digestion occur on the surface of small intestinal epithelial cells. To accommodate these processes, an extremely large mucosal surface area is required.

The absorptive surface area, referred to as the lumenal surface area of the small intestine, is approximately 250 square meters. This equates to the approximate size of a tennis court. The small intestine incorporates three features that account for its huge absorptive surface area:

1. The small intestine is not flat, but thrown into circular folds, which not only increase surface area, but aid in mixing the ingested food particles acting as baffles. These are called mucosal folds, also known as *Plicae*

2. The next feature is the *Villi*, whereby the mucosa forms multitudes of projections that protrude into the lumen and are covered with epithelial cells.

3. The final feature is where the lumenal plasma membrane of absorptive epithelial cells is studded with densely packed *Microvilli*.

The Microvillus border of intestinal epithelial cells is referred to as the brush border. The epithelial cells that mature into absorptive epithelial cells that cover the Villi are called Enteorcytes. These are the cells that take up and deliver into blood virtually all nutrients from the diet.

After the small intestine has absorbed as many nutrients as it can, the food particles are passed to the large intestine. The large intestine is more frequently referred to as the colon.

The Large Intestine / Colon

The large intestine is approximately 5 feet long and includes the appendix, cecum, colon, and rectum. It is the last part of the digestive system. The large intestine does not produce its own digestive enzymes, but contains huge numbers of bacteria which have the enzymes required for completion of the digestive process.

The first part of the large intestines is called the cecum. This is where the small intestines and large intestines join. The appendix is also found in this section.

The colon is the next part of the large intestines. The main function of the colon is to absorb water from the processed food residue that arrives after the nutrients have been absorbed in the small intestine. The colon constitutes the majority of the length of the large intestine and consists of the ascending, transverse and descending segments.

The Ascending Colon

The ascending colon is on the right side of the lower abdomen and ends at the hepatic flexure which is the beginning of the transverse colon. The ascending colon is the part of the colon with the largest diameter and the section that is most effective in absorbing water.

The Transverse Colon

The transverse colon extends from the splenic flexure to the hepatic flexure, across the abdomen from the right to the left. It follows a sagging course across, and in many people sag about three fourths of the way down to the naval.

The Descending Colon

The descending colon is in the left side of the lower abdomen, and can be felt whenever the abdominal muscles are fully relaxed. It hugs the left wall of the pelvis and reaches up to the splenic flexure, which is just under the left rib cage.

The Rectum

The last part of the large intestines is the rectum. The rectum is a reservoir for feces. Feces are stored here until it is convenient for their expulsion after which the sphincter muscles of the anus then relax.

Normal feces are roughly 75% water and 25% solids. The bulk of fecal solids are bacteria and undigested organic matter as well as fiber. The characteristic brown color of feces is due to chemicals produced by bacterial degradation of bilirubin, which is excreted in the bile. Fecal odor results from gases produced by bacterial metabolism.

In periods between meals, the colon is generally quiet and relaxed. Following a meal, colon activity increases significantly due to signals sent through the enteric nervous system. Several times each day the digestive process pushes feces into the rectum, which is usually empty. The stimulus for this process is call the gastrocolic reflex.

Distension of the rectum stimulates the defecation reflex. This is largely a spinal reflex mediated by the pelvic nerves. It results in reflex relaxation of the internal anal sphincter followed by voluntary relaxation of the external anal sphincter and defecation. Defecation can be prevented by voluntary constriction of the external sphincter. When this happens the rectum soon relaxes and the internal sphincter again contracts. The rectum will remain in this state until another movement of feces is forced into the rectum.

The Liver

The liver is a vital organ that performs many complex functions. Some of these functions are to convert food into chemicals necessary for life and growth; to manufacture and export important substances used by the rest of the body; to process drugs absorbed from the digestive tract into forms that are easier for the body to use; and to detoxify and excrete substances that otherwise would be poisonous to the body.

The liver plays a key role in converting food into essential chemicals of life. All of the blood that leaves the stomach and intestines must pass through the liver before reaching the rest of the body. The liver is thus strategically placed in the body to process nutrients and drugs absorbed from the digestive tract into forms that are easier for the rest of the body to use. The liver can be thought of as the body's refinery.

The liver helps the body by producing quick energy when it is needed by manufacturing new body proteins; preventing shortages in body fuel by storing certain vitamins, minerals, and sugars; regulating transport of fat stores; regulating blood clotting; aiding in the digestive process by producing bile; controlling the production and excretion of cholesterol; neutralizing and destroying poisonous substances; metabolizing alcohol; monitoring and maintaining the proper level of many chemicals and drugs in the blood; cleansing the blood and discharging waste products into the bile; maintaining hormone balance; serving as the main organ of blood formation before birth; helping the body resist infection by producing immune factors and by removing bacteria from the bloodstream; regenerating its own damaged tissue; and storing iron.

The liver also chemically modifies many drugs taken to treat diseases. These changes govern the drug's activity in the body.

The Pancreas

The pancreas is a small organ approximately six inches long and it is located in the upper abdomen and

34

connected to the small intestine. It is posterior in the body against the spine. It is this deep location that at times makes diagnosis of pancreatic disease difficult.

The pancreas is essential to the digestive process in two ways: First, it produces enzymes that help digest protein, fat and carbohydrates before they can be absorbed through the intestine; and, it makes islands of endocrine cells that produce insulin which regulate the use and storage of the body's main energy source, glucose or sugar.

The Gallbladder

The gallbladder is a four-inch sac with a muscular wall that is located under the liver. Here, about two to five cups of fluid are removed a day leaving a few tablespoons of concentrated bile. The gallbladder serves as a reservoir until bile is needed in the small intestine for digestion of fat. When food enters the small intestine, the hormone called CCK is released, signaling the gallbladder to contract. The force of the contraction propels the bile back through the common bile duct and then into the small intestine, where it emulsifies fatty molecules so that fat and the fat-absorbable vitamins A, D, E, and K can enter the blood stream through the intestinal lining.

Chapter 2

Basic Understanding of
Inflammatory Bowel Disease

Ulcerative colitis is an inflammatory disease of the large intestine. Ulcerative colitis causes inflammation and ulceration of the inner lining, or mucosa, of the colon and rectum. This inflammation may lead to bleeding in the bowel. Deeper ulceration through the entire wall of the intestine may lead to perforation of the bowel. The inflammation of ulcerative colitis is usually most severe in the rectal area with severity diminishing toward the area where the large and small intestines join. This diminishing of severity will vary from patient to patient.

Crohn's disease however, has significant deviations from this pattern and these deviations may be a clue to you and your doctor to suspect Crohn's disease instead of ulcerative colitis. Such deviations may include either skip areas and/or sparing of the rectum.

Skip areas are patches of healthy tissue separating segments of diseased tissue. These are common in Crohn's disease, but are rarely seen in patients with ulcerative colitis.

Inflammation of the rectum is called proctitis. Inflammation of the sigmoid colon, which is located just above the rectum, is called sigmoiditis. Inflammation involving the entire colon is called pancolitis. This inflammation causes the colon to empty frequently resulting in diarrhea. As the lining of the colon is destroyed, ulcers form releasing mucus, pus and blood and the affected areas may form abscesses or fistulas.

Fistulas are hollow tracts running from a part of one organ to other organs, adjacent loops of bowels, and/or the skin. They occur in Crohn's disease as a result of deep ulceration. Fistulas between loops of bowel can interfere with nutrient absorption. This is especially true for fistulas between the small and large bowel. Fistulas can also become infected forming abscesses.

Abscesses are collections of pus that may be accompanied by significant pain. Abscesses are not to be taken lightly because left untreated an abscess can become a life-threatening emergency. Simple treatment of abscesses resulting from fistulas can sometimes be accomplished by a procedure called incision and drainage, whereby an incision is made, through which the abscess is drained. However, this procedure does not deal with the underlying fistula, which caused the problem. In order to correct the cause and provide a more definitive treatment, a more elaborate procedure, known as a fistulectomy, is usually necessary. Fistulas are relatively common in Crohn's disease patients but are very rare in patients with ulcerative colitis.

Ileitis is Crohn's disease of the third part of the small intestine, known as the Ileum. Crohn's disease was thought at one time to affect only the Ileum so the term Ileitis was at one time synonymous with Crohn's disease. Now Ileitis simply refers to Crohn's disease of the Ileum.

Crohn's colitis results in Crohn's disease to affect part of or the entire colon and this form comprises about 20% of all cases of Crohn's disease. With this type of Crohn's disease, curious patterns are seen. In about 50% of these cases, lesions may be seen throughout one continuous section of the colon. In another 25%, skip areas are seen between multiple diseased areas. In the remaining 25%, the entire colon is involved, with no skip areas.

Ulcerative proctitis is a form of ulcerative colitis that affects only the rectum while Granulomatous colitis is another name for Crohn's disease that affects the colon.

Irritable Bowel Syndrome (IBS) is NOT a variant of ulcerative colitis or Crohn's disease. Ulcerative colitis and Crohn's disease are defined by the presence of inflammation in the intestine and are much more severe and dangerous than IBS. There is no inflammation in the intestine in IBS. IBS is also known as Functional Bowel Syndrome (FBS), Functional Bowel Disease (FBD) or spastic colon. Older terms for IBS are spastic or mucous colitis or even simply colitis. These terms are no longer used because they cause people to confuse IBS with ulcerative colitis. IBS is characterized by a variety of symptom patterns, which include diarrhea, constipation, alternating diarrhea/constipation and abdominal pain. Fever and/or bleeding are NOT features of IBS. IBS is much more common than Crohn's disease or ulcerative colitis and many people with symptoms of IBS do not seek medical attention.

It should be noted that some patients with Crohn's disease or ulcerative colitis could also have concurrent IBS.

Toxic mega colon is a severe dilation of the colon that occurs when inflammation spreads from the mucosa through the remaining layers of the colon. It is much more commonly a complication of ulcerative colitis than Crohn's disease though it can be seen occasionally in patients with Crohn's disease. If this condition exists, the colon becomes paralyzed which can lead to it eventually bursting. This condition is known as a perforation and is a dire medical emergency with a 30% mortality rate. Most patients with toxic mega colon require surgery.

Anyone with ulcerative colitis or Crohn's disease serious enough to be at risk for toxic mega colon should be hospitalized and closely monitored. Warning signs include abdominal pain/tenderness, abdominal distention, fever, large numbers of stools with obvious blood and a rapid (more than 100 / minute) pulse rate. Fortunately, this grave complication appears to be decreasing in frequency which probably reflects more effective treatment.

Use of certain drugs (opiates, opioids and/or anti-spasmodics) may intensify this complication. This is one of the reasons that patients who have ulcerative colitis or Crohn's disease should use narcotic relief type drugs very carefully.

Strictures are scar tissue from healed lesions that cause obstructions in the bowels resulting in the narrowing of the intestine. These strictures are seen in patients with Crohn's disease and usually develop in the small intestine and can result in severe cramps and vomiting. Strictures can also occur in the large intestine, but are much less common.

If the obstruction is due to a fibrous stricture then surgical resection may be necessary. If the obstruction is a consequence of inflammation, then it can usually be relieved by medical therapy such as steroids. In other patients it may be possible to clear some of these obstructions with a technique known as stricturoplasty. This technique attempts to expand the narrowed segment of the intestine.

In early Crohn's disease tiny inflamed ulcers form on the inner intestinal wall. Over time they may fuse and the intestinal wall takes on a "cobblestone" appearance. These are known as cobblestone ulcers.

Flexible sigmoidoscopy and colonoscopy are endoscopic procedures that allow doctors to examine the lining of the large intestine. In both procedures, the physician inserts a flexible tube known generically as an endoscope through the anus. (Crohn's patients always look forward to this procedure). The doctor is able to move this tube through the bowel to view the mucosal lining of the intestines. This also enables the doctor to take tiny tissue samples, known as biopsies, of the lining using a forceps passed through the endoscope.

A pathologist can then view these tissue samples under a microscope. Examination of these samples by a pathologist is particularly helpful in making the distinction between Crohn's disease and ulcerative colitis. They are also used for detecting the early evidence of cancerous change indicated by dysplasia, which is an abnormality of development, alteration in size, shape, and organization of adult cells.

A flexible sigmoidoscopy is a procedure done without sedation which examines the rectum, sigmoid colon and often a little bit more of the colon reaching as far as the splenic flexure which is the bend at which point the descending colon and transverse colon meet.

A Colonoscopy is a more elaborate procedure that is used to examine the entire length of the colon and is usually done with mild sedation. Both of these procedures will be discussed later.

In the treatment of Crohn's disease the use of Corticosteroids may be used. When using steroids over a long period of time, osteoporosis may occur. Osteoporosis is a disease that results in the destruction of bones causing them to become weak and much more likely to fracture. Without protection within the first six months of steroid therapy a person can lose 10 - 20% of bone mass.

As many as one in four of these people may eventually suffer a fracture as a result. Unlike osteoporosis associated with aging, steroid-induced osteoporosis can occur at any age, even in children.

The study of the frequency and distribution of diseases in the population is known as Epidemiology. Through years of studying patients with Crohn's disease and ulcerative colitis, epidemiologists have been able to gather enough information to know a good deal about the distribution of these diseases in the United States and Western Europe.

Studies showed that American Jews of European decent are four to five times more likely to develop Crohn's disease or ulcerative colitis than the general population, and although Crohn's disease and ulcerative colitis have long been considered a predominantly white disease, there has been a steady increase in reported cases of both Crohn's disease and ulcerative colitis among African Americans.

An HMO with approximately two million members reported over a six-year period, hospitalization rates of 10.2 per 100,000 for Whites and African Americans. This study also revealed that the prevalence rate among Hispanics and Asians were lower than that of whites and African Americans.

For reasons not yet understood by researchers, Crohn's disease and ulcerative colitis are largely diseases of the mainly the United States and Europe. Similarly, these diseases are reported to be more common in urban areas than in rural areas, and frequency of disease relapses appears to increase when populations move from developed to underdeveloped areas and vice versa.

Chapter 3

Crohn's Disease

Crohn's disease was given its name after our hero, Burrill B. Crohn (1884 - 1983). It was his name that was first in a three-author landmark paper published in 1932, which described the disease.

Crohn's disease is a very serious, chronic inflammatory disease of the digestive system. The disease primarily causes ulceration in the small intestine and the large intestine, but it can affect the digestive system anywhere between the mouth and the anus. Crohn's disease usually causes loss of appetite, weight loss, diarrhea, cramps, abdominal pain, joint pain, skin lesions, low-grade fever, and at times rectal bleeding. Once the disease begins it tends to be a chronic, recurrent condition with periods of remission followed by periods of relapse and flare of symptoms. These symptoms range from mild to severe. If treated properly, though, people with Crohn's disease can lead active and productive lives.

Children with the disease often suffer retarded physical growth.

The cause of Crohn's disease is unknown and there is no cure. Medication currently available only decreases inflammation and usually controls the symptoms. Crohn's disease behaves similarly to ulcerative colitis and it may be difficult to differentiate and incorrect diagnosis is common. These disorders are grouped together as inflammatory bowel disease (IBD), Crohn's disease being the most difficult to diagnose and treat.

Crohn's disease affects all layers of the intestine and there can be normal healthy bowel in between patches of diseased bowel. Ulcerative colitis affects only the innermost lining of the colon, known as the mucosa, in a continuous manner. Depending on where the involvement occurs, Crohn's disease may be referred to as Morbus Crohn's, Granulomatous enteritis, Regional enteritis, Terminal ileitis, or colitis.

To lessen the confusion, I will use the terms *Crohn's or Crohn's disease* to identify the disease wherever it occurs in the body.

Some scientists suspect that infection by certain bacteria such as strains of mycobacterium may be the cause of Crohn's disease. To date there has been no convincing evidence that the disease is caused by an infection. Crohn's disease is not contagious and although diet may affect the symptoms for patients with Crohn's disease, it appears unlikely that diet is responsible for the onset of the disease.

A research project fully supported and sponsored by the Crohn's and Colitis Foundation of America (CCFA) has been carried out in the fields of Immunology and Microbiology. Immunology is the study of the body's immune defense system and microbiology is the study of microscopic organisms.

The body's immune system and microscopic organisms have the power to cause this disease. Many scientists now believe that the interaction of an outside agent, such as a virus or bacterium, with the body's immune system may trigger the disease, or that such an agent may cause damage to the intestinal wall, initiating or accelerating the disease process.

For patients with Crohn's disease, the immune system seems to react actively to a variety of substances

43

and/or bacteria in the intestines, causing inflammation, bowel injury, and ulceration's. It is believed that the body's immune system is operating against some substances in the body, perhaps in the digestive tract itself, which the body recognizes as foreign. These foreign substances, known as antigens, may themselves cause the inflammation, or may stimulate the body's defenses to produce an inflammation that continues without control.

The body's immune system is composed of cells and proteins that normally protect the body from infections or other foreign invaders. In normal individuals no immune response will be directed against food, bacteria, and other substances in the intestines.

Scientists believe that an abnormally active immune system is genetically inherited. First-degree relatives of patients with Crohn's disease, such as brothers, sisters, sons and daughters, appear to be more likely to develop the disease.

Furthermore, certain chromosome markers have been found in patients with Crohn's disease. Chromosomes are components in the cells where all the genetic information of the body is stored.

Crohn's disease tends to run in families and studies have shown that about 20 - 25% of patients may have a close relative with either Crohn's or ulcerative colitis. There does not seem to be any clear-cut pattern to the family susceptibility but it does exist. Research actively continues in an attempt to establish a link to specific genes (DNA abnormalities) governing the disease transmission. At this time there is no way to predict which if any other family members will develop Crohn's disease.

Some Crohn's disease patients feel guilt and suffer severe depression with the thought that they have brought the illness upon themselves and may have caused problems both financially and emotionally to their families. These guilt feelings and the depression are usually the result of the patient's thinking that their Crohn's is caused by psychological factors. Some Crohn's patients feel that they somehow might have brought on this disease by not controlling their emotions. There is no basis or scientific proof for this way of thinking. Crohn's is not caused by emotions; however, the disease can have an impact on your emotions after diagnosis. Different people cope with physical illness in different ways. Some can cope with severe illness without an extraordinary emotional reaction while others experience emotional distress when they develop serious organic and chronic illnesses.

It is important to understand that the body and mind are inseparable and are interrelated in numerous and complex ways. It has been observed that flare-ups of Crohn's can occur at the time of stressful situations either physical or emotional. For instance, the first onset of Crohn's may occur at the time of an attack of a viral or other infectious illness. It also appears likely that some flare-ups of the disease can be triggered by nervous tension or by emotionally stressful life situations, such as divorce or a death in the family. This flare-up effect should be carefully separated from the primary cause of Crohn's.

There is nothing any patient could have done or avoided either emotionally or physically that would have prevented the onset of this disease. Guilt feelings and depression are completely unjustified and unwarranted but are very prevalent in patients with Crohn's. Indeed they make it more difficult to cope with the difficult physical burden that patients with Crohn's have to bear. It is therefore important for anyone with Crohn's, or any other chronic disease, to dispel such feelings.

Children and younger adults tend to be more severely affected by any chronic illness than individuals who have established a place in life for themselves and have learned to cope with adversity. Thus, the percentage of individuals who experience emotional problems in conjunction with Crohn's is somewhat higher among teenagers and young adults than among older adults.

The best way to effectively manage Crohn's at any age is to seek effective treatment. Most patients with Crohn's can be treated very well by means of anti-inflammatory drugs. There are numerous topical and oral medications that have been shown to be effective therapy. Your doctor, who is an expert in dealing with this disease, will decide which of these medications is best for you and your particular symptoms and condition.

Ideally you should accept your Crohn's realistically and without self-pity, guilt feelings, or blaming others for the illness. You should cope with this disease in a straightforward and matter-of-fact fashion because dealing with this disease like this will make it easier for friends and family to accept the illness as part of their relationship with you.

You should go about your life and daily activities as much as possible, follow your doctor's instructions, take your meds, eat right, exercise and maintain a positive attitude and optimistic outlook upon life.

If you have either partially or fully withdrawn from your normal life you should have the drive to get back to that life and its pleasures as soon as possible. You should not attempt to escape the realities of life by retiring to a sick bed. You should not use this illness to manipulate others in the family. Do for yourself as much as possible and only seek help from family members when necessary. It should be emphasized that following your doctor's advice with respect to clinical treatment is an important aspect of coping with this illness.

Chapter 4

Symptoms

For patients who have Crohn's disease, abdominal pain and diarrhea are often the earliest signs. The pain is primarily at or below the navel, also called the belly button. These symptoms often follow a meal or will occur during or shortly after engaging in activity that results in a high amount of stress. Loss of appetite, weight loss, joint pain, and low-grade fever are other common early signs of Crohn's disease. As the disease progresses symptoms can include sores in the anal area including skin tags mimicking hemorrhoids, fissures, fistulas, and abscesses.

Crohn's disease often involves the terminal ileum. This area is located adjacent to the appendix and results in right-sided abdominal pain and tenderness mimicking appendicitis. The pain can also be cramp-like in nature and may indicate obstruction of the bowel. As scarring and inflammation progresses it results in narrowing of the bowel.

Obstruction may occur acutely by the eating a poorly digestible fruit or vegetables that plug up the already narrowed segment of the intestine. Symptoms of obstruction include cramping, abdominal pain, abdominal distention, nausea and vomiting.

Diarrhea is also common and may be due to partial bowel obstruction, excessive growth of bacteria in the small bowel, poor absorption of nutrients and bile acids as well as inflammation of the large intestine.

Crohn's disease may cause the intestines to contain blood and rectal bleeding is common while massive bleeding, known as hemorrhaging, is rare.

Approximately one third of patients with Crohn's disease have symptoms involving the anal area.

Other symptoms that may be experienced are abdominal mass, abdominal sounds such as a gurgling or splashing sound heard over the intestine known as borgorygmus; clubbing of the fingers or toes, foul smelling and/or bloody stools, tenesmus, painful stools, incontinence, swollen gums, constipation and abdominal fullness.

Crohn's disease patients may experience constipation during periods of active disease. This can result from a partial obstruction usually of the small intestine. It can also be a consequence of inflammation of the rectum whereby the colon has a nervous reaction and stasis, or maintenance, of the stool occurs higher in the colon.

Inflammation can affect nerves in such a way as to make the patient feel that there is stool present ready to be evacuated when there actually is not. This is a symptom known as tenesmus. This feeling of urgency to pass stool is a frequent consequence of inflammation of the rectum. Inability to retain stool should cause an extreme sense of urgency. It is important to bring these symptoms to the attention of your doctor. These may improve dramatically with appropriate local therapy.

Constipation is passage of small amounts of hard, dry bowel movements, usually fewer than three times a week. People who are constipated may find it difficult and painful to have a bowel movement. Other symptoms of constipation include feeling bloated, uncomfortable, and sluggish.

Many people think they are constipated when in fact their bowel movements are regular. For example, some

49

people believe they are constipated, or irregular, if they do not have a bowel movement every day. Keep in mind there is no right number of daily or weekly bowel movements. Normal may be three times a day or three times a week depending on the person. Also, some people naturally have firmer stools.

At one time or another almost everyone gets constipated. Poor diet and lack of exercise are usually the causes. In most cases, constipation is temporary and not serious. Understanding causes, prevention, and treatment will help most people find relief.

Pain usually results from intestinal cramping or inflammation, causing your body to reflex and irritate the nerves and muscles that control intestinal contractions. Pain may also indicate the presence of severe inflammation or the development of a complication such as an abscess or a perforation of the intestinal wall. Generally, new pain or a significant change in the character of pain should be brought to the attention of your doctor.

The pain that a Crohn's disease patient often feels is in the lower right area of the abdomen. That usually indicates inflammation of the terminal ileum. However, location and intensity of abdominal pain vary from patient to patient, depending upon the location of the disease in the affected tissues.

Because of a phenomenon known as referred pain or ghost pain, the location where pain is produced may not be the same as the location where it is actually experienced.

Chapter 5

Complications

Complications of Crohn's disease may be occur in the intestines (intestinal/local) or occur in areas unrelated to the intestines (extra-intestinal/systemic). Complications are usually categorized as local or systemic. The term local refers to a complication involving the digestive system itself. The term systemic refers to complications involving other organs or complications that affect the patient as a whole.

The list of complications is a laundry list of problems that a Crohn's disease patient can and probably will experience. Some of the complications are directly caused by the Crohn's disease itself. Treatment and medications cause some and the patients own doing brings on other complications. Regardless of what the source of the complication is, it must be addressed and resolved as soon as the symptoms occur.

If a condition is left untreated, it most likely will cause other complications, which in turn causes the need for more medications, which in turn causes more complications ... well, you get my drift.

Simply put, you cannot ignore your body when it tells you that something is wrong.

Intestinal (local) Complications

Intestinal complications occur within the digestive system and include bowel obstruction, bowel perforation, formation abscesses, fistulae, cancer of the bowel, and intestinal hemorrhage. Progressive scarring and inflammation of the bowel causes narrowing. Sometimes, obstruction can be acutely caused by the ingestion of poorly digestible fruit or vegetables that plug the already narrowed segment of the intestine. Symptoms of obstruction include cramps, abdominal pain, abdominal distention or enlargement, nausea and vomiting.

If an inflammatory ulcer appears and burrows through the bowel wall, it may tunnel into adjacent structures. If the ulcer tract reaches an adjacent empty space inside the abdomen, an abscess is formed. Patients with abdominal abscesses may develop spiking fevers and tender abdominal masses.

When the ulcer burrows into an adjacent organ, a fistula, or tube, is formed. When a fistula, or tube, develops between the bowel and the bladder, the patient can develop recurrent urinary infections, and passage of air and feces in the urine. A fistula can also occur between the intestine and the skin, leading to the discharge of pus or mucus through a small painful opening on the skin of the abdomen.

Massive dilatation of the colon (toxic mega colon) and rupture of the intestine are potentially life-threatening complications. Both conditions generally require surgery. Fortunately these two complications are rare.

Recent data suggest that there is an increased risk of cancer of the small intestines and the colon for patients with long-standing Crohn's disease. Cancer of the small intestine is very rare; although, cancer of the colon occurs more frequently than previously thought.

Extra-intestinal (systemic) Complications

Extra-intestinal complications occur outside the digestive system. These complications include tender, raised, reddish skin nodules (erythema nodosum), and an ulcerating skin condition generally found around the ankles (pyoderma gangrenosum), and inflammation of the following areas the joints (sacroiliac joint arthritis), stiffness of the spine (ankylosing spondylitis), the eyes (uveitis, episceritis and conjunctivitis), the liver (hepatitis), and the bile ducts (sclerosing cholangitis) that drain the liver. The most common complication outside the digestive tract is joint pain.

Some consider the extra-intestinal complications to be secondary to the primary disease, while others see both the extra-intestinal complications and the primary disease as symptoms of the overall Crohn's condition. Those of us who experienced any of the extra-intestinal complications from Crohn's disease will agree with the latter. We know that the problems caused by these complications are sometimes severe and in and of themselves can cause tremendous health problems, up to and becoming bed ridden.

Additional Complications

Other complications that can occur are fatigue, which is one of the most common complications. Fever usually indicates an active disease and/or a complication such as an abscess. Severe diarrhea, blood loss or infection can lead to rapid heartbeat and a drop in blood pressure. Continued loss of small amounts of blood in the stool that may not be visible and may lead to anemia, which is a reduced blood count. This may be the cause of fatigue in Crohn's patients.

By far the most concerning complication that Crohn's disease patients face is the risk of cancer. For patients who have had Crohn's disease longer than ten years, the risk of colon cancer is greater than that for comparable people without the disease. There is data that suggests a risk of 5 - 10% at that point increasing to a range between 15 and 40% after thirty years. These numbers depend upon the particular study you wish to consider.

Studies also show that if only the rectum and lower colon are involved, the risk of cancer does not appear to be significantly increased. Patients that exhibit dysplasia are at much higher risk. Other cancers, such as lymphoma or carcinoma of the small intestine or anus, may be slightly more common in Crohn's patients, but the risk is not high.

After a Crohn's patient reaches the 7 – 8 year timeframe with the disease, in which the disease involves more than the rectum and sigmoid colon or extensive Crohn's disease, then the consensus of the medical opinion is that the patient should have a regular screening colonoscopy to look for evidence of dysplasia. This colonoscopy should be performed yearly or every other year and if dysplasia is found, then the safest option is for a colectomy to be performed.

Other factors affecting the development of colon cancer appear that Crohn's patients who have sclerosing cholangitis may be at a greater risk of developing colon cancer. Because of that greater risk, particular attention to regular screening should be done with these patients.

There is also some data suggesting that low folic acid levels may affect the development of colon cancer in Crohn's patients.

There are some ways to reduce the risk of developing colon cancer. The only certain way eliminate the risk of colon cancer is to have a colectomy and have the colon removed surgically. There is some circumstantial evidence that taking 5-ASA drugs, such as azulfidine, might reduce the risk of colon cancer. There is also some data that eating a diet rich in fruit and vegetables and low in red meat is associated with a reduced risk of colon cancer in people without colitis. Regular exercise also seems to be associated with a reduced risk of colon cancer. These associations may also be true for Crohn's patients but they have not been studied.

These strategies do not guarantee that cancer can be avoided but seems to significantly increase the probability that will not be life threatening if and when it is detected.

Small Bowel Obstruction

Small bowel obstruction occurs when something causes the small bowel to be blocked and material can't pass through the bowel. The small bowel can be obstructed for a number of reasons, the most common being previous surgery. Whenever the abdominal cavity is opened, there is a possibility of adhesions, which are a reaction of normal tissue to injury or decreased blood supply. The result is that there may be attachments of the bowel to the abdominal wall or to other structures such as the liver or spleen. This intra abdominal scarring can cause pain, constipation, diarrhea, and sometimes obstruction. The adhesions can be so severe that as they form, the bowel is completely blocked. When this occurs it is like tying a rope around the bowel.

The two other most common causes of bowel obstruction are entrapment in hernias, usually inguinal hernias, and cancer. Bowel obstruction is usually not an acute process though it may present with fairly sudden onset of nausea, vomiting, and abdominal pain. Most Crohn's patients with this condition will present a history of insidious abdominal cramping and intermittent nausea well before the actual acute episode occurs.

The most common symptoms of a blockage are nausea, vomiting, loss of appetite, cramping abdominal pain and at the onset of a blockage the patient usually will not have bowel movements for a few days. An area of adhesions may aggravate into a bowel obstruction by irritation or inflammation, known as gastroenteritis. There may be susceptibility to a urinary tract infection if the patient is predisposed to adhesions. Not all patients form adhesions with surgery and in rare cases adhesions can form without any previous surgery.

Once a Crohn's patient develops symptoms of a bowel obstruction, a simple abdominal X-ray usually confirms the diagnosis. An experienced physician can determine from the film whether there is an actual obstruction, or whether the bowel function is an intestinal motility, known as an ileus.

The initial treatment for a suspected obstruction is bowel test, which usually means the insertion of a Nasogastric (NG) tube through the anus. Though this treatment is not particularly pleasant, it is most definitely preferable to surgery.

If your body fails to clear the obstruction in 24 - 48 hours or you develop abdominal pain, fever, or increasing white blood count, then surgery will most likely be required. In about 70% of patients, the obstruction will clear with conservative, non-surgical care.

The standard approach to bowel obstruction has always been an exploratory laparotomy but a bowel obstruction can often be evaluated and treated minimally invasive laparoscopic techniques. When a patient can be cured with laparoscopy the formation of adhesions appears to be reduced compared to an exploratory laparotomy. The risk of recurrence is also reduced.

Currently, there is no proven method to reduce intrabdominal adhesions. While some patients get dense adhesions following a surgical procedure, others have the exact same procedure and will have none at all.

There is continuing research to find prevention for postoperative adhesions.

Intestinal pseudo-obstruction

Intestinal pseudo-obstruction, which is a false blockage of the bowel, is a condition that causes symptoms like those of a bowel obstruction. This condition is discovered when the intestines are examined and no obstruction is found. The symptoms of intestinal pseudo-obstruction are caused by a problem in how the muscles and nerves in the intestines work.

Symptoms of pseudo-obstruction include cramps, stomach pain, nausea, vomiting, bloating, fewer bowel movements than usual, and loose stools. Over time, pseudo-obstruction can cause bacterial infections, malnutrition, and muscle problems in other parts of the body. Some patients with intestinal pseudo-obstruction also have bladder problems.

Some diseases that affect muscles and nerves can cause symptoms of pseudo-obstruction. Medications that affect muscles and nerves such as opiates and antidepressants might also cause secondary pseudo-obstruction.

In order to diagnose this condition, your doctor will take a complete medical history, do a physical exam, and take x-rays. The main treatment is intravenous feeding to prevent malnutrition and antibiotics to treat bacterial infections. This also allows the digestive system, especially the bowels, to rest. Medication may also be given to help with intestinal muscle problems and in severe cases, surgery to remove part of the intestines might be necessary.

Systemic Effects on the Liver

Primary Sclerosing Cholangitis

Although rare, Primary Sclerosing Cholangitis is a disease in which the bile ducts inside and outside the liver become narrowed due to inflammation and scarring. This causes bile to accumulate in the liver and can result in damage to liver cells. Although the exact cause of Primary Sclerosing Cholangitis is unknown, genetic and immunologic factors appear to play a role. Primary Sclerosing Cholangitis has been considered a rare disease, but recent studies suggest that it is more common than previously thought. It may occur alone, but approximately 70% of patients have associated inflammatory bowel disease, particularly ulcerative colitis.

Primary Sclerosing Cholangitis is more common in men than women. Initially, many individuals have no symptoms and the disease is detected because of abnormal laboratory test results, particularly an enzyme test called alkaline phosphates. It usually begins in the patients' 30s, 40s, and 50s, and is commonly associated with fatigue, itching and jaundice. Episodes of fever and chills from superimposed infection in the bile ducts occasionally occur and can be distressing symptoms.

The diagnosis of Primary Sclerosing Cholangitis is made by Cholangiography, an X-ray test involving injection of dye into the bile ducts. This is usually accomplished by an endoscopic procedure called Endoscopic Retrograde Cholangiopancreatography, known as ECRP, but also may be done radiologically or surgically.

The course of the disease is unpredictable for the patient, but is generally progresses slowly. The patient may have the disease for many years before symptoms develop and symptoms may persist at a stable level, intermittent, or progress gradually. Liver failure may occur after 7 - 15 years of disease. In some patients, this time can be extended even longer. Approximately 10% of patients who have the disease on a longstanding basis may develop a superimposed tumor of the bile ducts called cholangiocarcinoma.

There is currently no specific treatment for Primary Sclerosing Cholangitis. Research is under way to determine the effectiveness of various medications. The symptoms of Primary Sclerosing Cholangitis often respond effectively to medications that control itching. In the case of recurrent infections antibiotics are given. Vitamins are taken to replace those that are deficient because of the disease. In some instances, endoscopic, radiological, or surgical techniques may be employed to open major blockages in the common bile duct and improve bile flow. When progressive liver failure occurs in spite of these measures, liver transplantation may be required. Liver transplant has a survival rate of 75% or more. There is usually a good quality of life after recovery.

Hepatitis

Hepatitis is the general name for liver inflammation. Symptoms of hepatitis vary depending on the specific cause of the illness (virus, drug-related, toxin, etc.) and how much liver damage has been done. In mild cases, many patients either are asymptomatic, which means they have no symptoms. Conversely, they have flu like symptoms which may include fever, a generally tired or ill feeling, loss of appetite, nausea and vomiting, diarrhea, and muscle aches.

With more significant liver inflammation, liver chemicals can build up in the blood and urine, causing the following symptoms: jaundice, which is a yellow tint to the skin and whites of the eyes; bad breath or a

59

bitter taste in the mouth; dark tea-colored urine or light clay-colored stools. There also can be pain or tenderness in the area of the liver, which is located in the upper-right side of the abdomen near the lower-front ribs.

Your doctor will note your specific symptoms of hepatitis. On physical examination, your doctor will look for a yellowish tint to your skin and the whites of your eyes, and also will examine your abdomen for tenderness and swelling in the liver area.

After performing a physical examination, your doctor will have blood tests performed to confirm the diagnosis of hepatitis. These blood tests typically measure levels of liver chemicals, as well as levels of antibodies or antigens related to the hepatitis viruses. In some cases, your doctor also may need to order other special tests, including urine tests, laboratory cultures, stool samples, blood coagulation tests, an ultrasound or Computerized Tomography Scan, known as a CT Scan.

The duration of hepatitis varies depending on the type of hepatitis, as well as the age and basic health of the patient. For example, most previously healthy adults and children who develop hepatitis A usually recover completely. This recovery usually takes about one month. About 5% of adults with acute hepatitis A will go on to develop chronic hepatitis B infection. The rate is much higher for babies and young children. A small percentage of these patients eventually will develop cirrhosis or liver cancer. Up to 80% of those infected with hepatitis C will develop chronic infection, and about 20 - 30% of these patients will develop cirrhosis or liver cancer.

Call your doctor if you have symptoms of hepatitis, or if you believe that you have been exposed to someone with hepatitis. A person may be especially susceptible if they are planning to travel to a foreign country. If you travel outside the country, make sure to ask your doctor about your need for hepatitis immunization before your trip.

Most patients with either hepatitis A or B recover spontaneously. Up to 85% of those with hepatitis C, and a smaller number of those with hepatitis B, develop chronic hepatitis. Some patients with hepatitis B become lifelong carriers of the illness and can spread the hepatitis infection to others. Patients with chronic hepatitis C also are infectious usually spreading the virus through blood-to-blood contact.

Cirrhosis

Cirrhosis is a disease in which normal liver cells are replaced by scar tissue that interferes with all of the functions of the liver. In extreme cases, damage is so severe that the only solution is a transplant. Cirrhosis is the eighth leading cause of death by disease in the United States, killing approximately 25,000 people each year. It impairs thousands of other people as the liver gradually loses its ability to function.

Cirrhosis has many causes. In the United States and Europe, the most common causes are excessive alcohol use and chronic infection with the hepatitis C virus.

Alcoholic cirrhosis tends to develop after a decade or more of heavy drinking, although it is possible for social drinkers to have cirrhosis. Alcohol has a toxic effect on liver cells. It is not known why some people are more prone to adverse reactions than others, but women in particular are at greater risk for cirrhosis, even when they consume less alcohol than men.

Rarer causes of cirrhosis include autoimmune diseases that attack the bile ducts or liver cells, severe reactions to prescription drugs, prolonged exposure to environmental toxins, infections from bacteria and parasites usually found in the tropics and repeated episodes of heart failure with liver congestion.

Another cause is nonalcoholic steatohepatitis (NASH), which causes fat to build up in the liver and produces scarring.

In its early stages, cirrhosis often has no symptoms. But as liver cells die, the organ makes less of the proteins that regulate fluid retention and blood clotting and loses its ability to metabolize the pigment bilirubin. The resulting symptoms and complications include fatigue, loss of appetite, nausea and vomiting, weakness, weight loss, fluid accumulation in the legs called edema, fluid accumulation in the abdomen called ascites, increased bleeding and bruising, jaundice and itching.

As damage increases, the liver fails to detoxify the blood and it becomes less able to metabolize many medications which magnifies their effects. Eventually toxins build up in the brain. These changes may produce increased sensitivity to drugs, personality and behavioral changes, including confusion, neglect of appearance, forgetfulness, trouble concentrating or changes in sleep habits, loss of consciousness, coma and eventually death.

Scarring also impedes blood flow and increases pressure in the portal vein, which is a condition called portal hypertension. Blood vessels in the stomach and esophagus swell and the body creates new ones in an attempt to bypass the liver. These vessels, called varices, have very thin walls. If one bursts, the resulting hemorrhage can cause death in a matter of hours. *If you are vomiting blood, go to the emergency room immediately.*

Blood tests may be ordered to look for evidence of a buildup of toxins or reduced levels of essential substances made by the liver. The liver may be viewed using a CT Scan, ultrasound or a harmless radioactive highlighting substance called a radioisotope.

Cirrhosis may also be confirmed through a biopsy, in which a tiny sample of liver tissue is removed and then examined for scarring and damage to cells.

Cirrhosis is a progressive disease that has no cure, but damage in many cases may be halted or slowed down with treatment or changes in behavior.

The most important step you can take to prevent cirrhosis is to avoid excessive drinking. It is best to consume an average of no more than two alcoholic drinks a day for men or one drink a day for women. If you have chronic hepatitis or other liver problems, avoid alcohol completely. Regardless of the cause, all cirrhosis patients should abstain from alcohol and use caution in taking medications that can exacerbate liver disease, including over-the-counter acetaminophen such as Tylenol.

Treatment for cirrhosis varies depending on the cause and stage of the disease. Because liver damage can only be reversed to a certain point, the aim of all treatment is to keep the disease from getting worse and to reduce complications.

Much of the treatment is directed at complications. Your doctor may recommend a low-sodium diet or diuretics to reduce fluid in the body. Laxatives may hasten the removal of toxins. Medications can be prescribed for itching and infections. Blood pressure medicines may help to control portal hypertension.

Bleeding varices can be treated in several ways. They may be tied off with a rubber band or compressed with an inflated balloon to stop the bleeding. In sclerotherapy, the blood vessel is injected with a chemical that causes it to scar and wither away.

Transjugular intrahepatic portosystemic shunt (TIPS) involves creating a new passageway for blood by inserting a tube, or shunt, through the scarred liver to take pressure off the varices. Drugs also may be prescribed to reduce the likelihood of bleeding or rebleeding.

If the liver is too scarred to function, a transplant is the only treatment. Approximately 80 - 90% of patients survive liver transplantation. Overall, long-term survival rates have improved because of drugs such as Cyclosporine that suppress the immune system to keep it from attacking the new liver.

See your doctor if you have any of the symptoms of cirrhosis, particularly if you are a heavy drinker or have chronic hepatitis. *If you are vomiting blood, go to the emergency room immediately.* Patients who already have been diagnosed with cirrhosis should see a doctor promptly if symptoms get worse or if they become disoriented or develop a fever or abdominal pain.

Treatment leads to improvement in most cases when the disease is discovered in its earlier stages. Most patients are able to live a normal life for many years. The outlook is less favorable if liver damage is extensive or if someone with alcoholic cirrhosis does not stop drinking. Either bleeding or loss of brain function can cause death in cirrhosis patients. Patients with cirrhosis are more likely to develop serious infections and are susceptible to kidney dysfunction and failure.

Liver Cancer

Cancer within the liver that originates in that organ is called primary liver cancer. The American Cancer Society estimates that about 14,500 Americans will die from primary liver cancer in 2002, most of them over the age of 40. In the United States, liver cancer is about twice as common in men as in women.

Although relatively rare in the United States and Europe, primary liver cancer is common in other countries. In fact it is the most common solid tumor worldwide with over one million cases diagnosed each year. This type of cancer is particularly common in areas with a high incidence of viral hepatitis, namely in some parts of Africa and Asia. In the United States most tumors within the liver began in other organs, such as the lung, breast or colon, and spread to the liver. These cancers are not truly liver cancer, and should be treated differently.

Metastatic Liver Cancer

When cancer spreads to the liver from other organs, it is called liver metastases. Liver metastases are tumor growths that begin in other organs and spread to the liver, where they implant and grow. These tumors are sometimes called secondary liver cancer. Secondary liver cancer is much more common than primary liver cancer in the United States.

The most common primary cancers that spread to the liver are cancers of the colon, rectum, lung, breast, pancreas and stomach. When cancer spreads from its primary origin, the new tumor has the same kind of cancer cells and the same name as the primary cancer. For example, if colon cancer spreads to the liver, the cancer cells in the liver are colon-cancer cells, and the disease is called metastatic colon cancer. It is not primary liver cancer.

The liver is the most common site of metastatic disease and unfortunately, the reason for this is not clear. Many researchers believe that this organ has high blood flow and provides sort of a fertile soil for the attachment and growth of metastatic cancer cells.

When liver metastases are isolated or confined to part of the liver, aggressive surgical therapy occasionally can result in significant prolongation in survival. In patients with metastatic colorectal cancer, successful removal of limited numbers of metastases can result in a 5 year survival rate of about 30%. In a healthy liver, up to 70% of the liver can be resected with success, and the liver will regenerate back to normal size over time.

Primary Liver Cancer

Primary liver cancer is an aggressive and often a fatal type of cancer, with most patients not living longer than six months after diagnosis. One reason is that treatment options are limited; another reason is that the disease is rarely diagnosed in its early stages. Liver cancer can produce signs and symptoms but these usually do not appear until the later stages of the disease. At this time there are no accurate and efficient screening tests that have proven beneficial in the United States. Those who have hepatitis B, hepatitis C or cirrhosis of the liver from other causes have a higher risk of developing primary liver cancer.

There are ways to limit the risk of developing liver cancer. Most liver cancer in the United States is caused by chronic viral hepatitis, so reducing the risk of acquiring hepatitis B or hepatitis C can lower the risk of liver cancer. The hepatitis B vaccine can lower the risk of infection with this virus. Alcohol use and resulting cirrhosis of the liver also are risk factors for liver cancer, so limiting alcohol intake to one or two drinks per day can also reduce the risk of liver cancer.

The four main types of primary liver cancer are:

- Hepatocellular Carcinoma
- Cholangiocarcinoma
- Angiosarcoma
- Hepatoblastoma.

Hepatocellular carcinoma

Hepatocellular carcinoma, also called Hepatoma or HCC, is the most common type of primary liver cancer. In the United States, HCC accounts for about 84% of primary liver cancers. Its incidence worldwide varies widely by region, but it is as high as 500 cases per 100,000 people in some parts of Africa and Asia. HCC develops from damaged hepatocytes, the main type of liver cell, and exhibits an aggressive behavior.

The exact cause of HCC is unknown, but contributing factors include chronic liver diseases such as hepatitis B, hepatitis C, alcoholic cirrhosis and hemochromatosis, certain chemicals, and aflatoxin, which is a substance found in foods in parts of Asia and Africa. Worldwide, hepatitis B and C are the leading causes of HCC. Some experts believe that hepatitis C could be responsible for the majority of liver cancer cases in the United States.

Usually patients with HCC have no symptoms until the cancer is quite advanced. When symptoms do develop they can include abdominal pain or tenderness, nausea, loss of appetite, and weight loss. Aggressive surgery can be an option for treatment particularly if the liver is otherwise relatively healthy. If surgery is successful, five-year survival rates of 20 - 40% are seen.

Cholangiocarcinoma

Cholangiocarcinoma, or bile-duct cancer, develops within the liver in small bile ducts and is responsible for about 13% of primary liver cancers in the United States. The worldwide incidence of this cancer is 5 cases out of 100,000 people. A person's risk of this type of liver cancer is increased if there is a history of gallstones, gallbladder inflammation, chronic ulcerative colitis, or a chronic infection with some types of parasites seen in Asia.

The most common symptom at the time of diagnosis is jaundice. Other typical signs and symptoms include right upper-abdominal pain, weight loss, fever, loss of appetite, itching and stools that are clay colored.

One type of Cholangiocarcinoma, known as a Klatskin tumor, tends to produce jaundice without abdominal pain. This tumor starts in the area where the bile ducts exit the liver, before they reach the gallbladder.

Several tests can be performed to show a tumor or an obstruction in the bile duct. The most commonly used tests are ultrasounds, CT Scans, Magnetic Resonance Imaging scans, known as MRI's, and ECRP.

Surgical removal is attempted when possible, however; because of their size, location or both, most cholangiocarcinomas cannot be completely removed by surgery.

Stint placement or surgery to bypass bile ducts blocked by the cancer sometimes can relieve symptoms of this liver cancer. Radiation therapy may be beneficial, but chemotherapy has not been shown to be as effective. If a tumor can be removed surgically, the chances of long-term cure are between 15 and 40%.

Angiosarcoma,

Angiosarcoma, also called Hemangiosarcoma, is a very rare form of liver cancer that begins in the blood vessels of the liver. Angiosarcomas, which are often associated with exposure to vinyl chloride and arsenic, grow rapidly and are usually too widespread to be removed by the time they are diagnosed.

Chemotherapy and radiation therapies are usually not effective, and most patients survive less than six months.

Hepatoblastoma

Hepatoblastoma is also a rare type of liver cancer that usually is found in children younger than 4 years. Treatment is, with or without chemotherapy, surgical resection. The cure rate can be as high as 70% with aggressive therapy.

There are also several types of benign liver tumors that can form in the liver. These tumors, although considered cancer, they are not malignant and are caused by different risk factors than malignant tumors.

Hemangiomas

Hemangiomas is the most common type of benign liver tumor. They are abnormally dense collections of capillaries, which are small, dilated blood vessels. Most hemangiomas of the liver do not cause any symptoms, but if the tumor becomes large enough, it may cause pain by stretching the liver capsule.

A CT Scan or an MRI can be used to detect Hemangiomas. Hemangiomas rarely require any treatment unless they are symptomatic and surgical removal is the treatment of choice.

Other Liver Cancer / Tumor Disorders

Hepatic adenomas

These are rare tumors that begin from hepatocytes, which is the main type of liver cell. Hepatic adenomas are more common in women than in men. Researchers

69

believe that a woman's risk of developing a hepatic adenoma increases with long-term use of oral contraceptives. Most hepatic adenomas do not cause any symptoms but some cause abdominal pain or a mass in the abdomen. These tumors do not spread, but they can rupture and cause internal bleeding. They are also thought to have a potential for transforming into a malignant, cancerous tumor. In most cases, surgical resection is the recommended treatment for all Hepatic adenomas.

Focal nodular hyperplasia

This is a rare growth of the liver and is similar to a tumor. It can include liver cells, connective tissues and bile-duct cells. Focal nodular hyperplasia is more common in women than in men and a woman's risk of developing focal nodular hyperplasia is increased by long-term use of oral contraceptives. This condition rarely causes symptoms, and surgical therapy is rarely indicated unless the diagnosis is in question.

Hemochromatosis

Hemochromatosis is a common genetic disorder in which increased amounts of iron are absorbed from the digestive tract. This excess iron is deposited in the tissues and organs of the body where it may become toxic and cause damage.

Hemochromatosis occurs most often in people of northern European ancestry, especially those of Scottish, Irish or English decent, and affects up to one in 250 people in the United States. Hemochromatosis is most commonly diagnosed in those between ages 40 and 60. In women, it is usually diagnosed after menopause.

The early symptoms of hemochromatosis are nonspecific and can vary widely and include weakness, weight loss, joint pain, abdominal pain, heart palpitations, irritability, impotence, depression and loss of body hair.

As the condition progresses, the skin may take on a bronze or yellowish color. Progressive deposits of iron in the tissues and organs may lead to organ failure, especially cirrhosis of liver, a condition that may cause confusion, bleeding, fluid accumulation in the legs and abdomen, black or bloody stools, and jaundice. Deposits of iron in the heart may cause shortness of breath and an irregular heartbeat. If the pancreas is involved, you may also develop diabetes, which may lead to frequent urination and excessive thirst.

A liver biopsy is often recommended to confirm the diagnosis. In this procedure the patient receives a local anesthetic, and a small piece of tissue from the liver is removed for analysis. Some experts now recommend screening all adults for this disorder, regardless of symptoms. Testing is available for two of the more common genes associated with this disorder which is found in up to 90% of people with Hemochromatosis. It should be noted however, not all carriers of the genes develop the disease.

Hemochromatosis is a lifelong condition and as with other conditions that causes liver damage, vaccination for hepatitis A and B should be considered.

There is no way to prevent Hemochromatosis because the disorder is inherited. One may prevent the complications of the disease, including cirrhosis, arthritis, heart failure and diabetes, by early detection and treatment. Avoiding supplemental iron (as in vitamins) and high doses of vitamin C (which frees iron to deposit in the tissues) may also help prevent complications of iron overload.

The traditional treatment for Hemochromatosis is periodic Phlebotomy, known as removal of blood. This is similar to the task of blood donation. Blood may be removed at variable intervals, up to once a week, until iron levels are normalized. Thereafter, maintenance Phlebotomy is usually needed about every 2 - 4 months to keep iron levels in the blood at an acceptable level. The patient's blood count will be monitored to make sure that too much blood is not being removed. Too much blood loss can lead to anemia. Some dietary modifications may also be suggested.

Call your doctor if you have a family history of Hemochromatosis or are starting to experience any of the symptoms of the disease. Make sure your Doctor checks you for this condition when you see him.

With early diagnosis and treatment, the serious consequences of iron overload in the body can be avoided. Unfortunately, once tissue damage has developed, problems related to that damage, such as arthritis or diabetes, are usually chronic. A liver transplant is sometimes necessary for people with advanced liver failure, and people with hemochromatosis and cirrhosis of the liver have an increased incidence of Hepatoma.

Systemic Effects of the Skin

Erythema nodosum

Erythema nodosum is characterized by tender, red bumps, called nodules, usually found on the shins. Quite often Erythema nodosum is not a separate disease but rather a sign of some other disease or sensitivity to a drug. Erythema nodosum is most common in women between the ages of 20 and 30 but can occur in anyone at any age.

There are several diseases that can cause Erythema nodosum. Among them are Streptococcal infections, Sarcoidosis, which is inflammation of the lymph nodes and other organs, leprosy, Coccidioidomycosis, which is an infection of the upper respiratory tract and lungs, Histoplasmosis, which is an infectious pulmonary disease, tuberculosis, psittacosis, which is a flu-like disease, Lymphogranuloma venereum infection, cat-scratch disease, and ulcerative colitis.

Some drugs that can cause Erythema nodosum are antibiotics containing sulfa, bromides, iodides and oral contraceptives.

Besides the painful nodules on the shins, Erythema nodosum sufferers also can experience fever, joint pain and enlarged lymph nodes in the chest.

A biopsy of a bump is the only way to accurately diagnose Erythema nodosum. If the biopsy proves that the patient has Erythema nodosum, the doctor will then try to determine the cause of the condition. This may involve lab work and skin tests. The exact cause can not always be identified but drug-caused Erythema nodosum can usually be diagnosed by careful elimination of the drug causing it.

Specific treatment for Erythema nodosum will be determined by your physician based on the cause of the disorder and may include antibiotics, treatment of underlying cause, bed rest to relieve pain, aspirin; Corticosteroids or an aspirin like drug called Indocin. A warm soapy wash cloth held over the area for 30 minutes three to four times a day often speeds up the healing process.

Erythema nodosum is not dangerous or contagious and it usually goes away after the underlying cause of the condition is found.

Pyoderma gangrenosum

Pyoderma gangrenosum is a chronic ulcerative disease of the skin characterized by deep ulcers with extensive necrosis around the edges of the lesions with ragged bluish-red overhanging edges. The ulcers generally begin as a small pustule or a tender nodule that enlarges and subsequently ulcerates. The lesions often occur at sites of trauma and the disease may occur alone or in conjunction with a variety of underlying disorders. It is associated with systemic diseases in at least 50% of affected patients, in particular, patients with ulcerative colitis or Crohn's disease, rheumatoid-like arthritis, liver disease, abnormal increases in antibody production, known as monoclonal gammopathies, and hematologic cancers.

There are two primary variants of Pyoderma gangrenosum. The first variant is the classic ulceration, which is usually observed on the legs. The second variation is a more superficial variant known as atypical Pyoderma gangrenosum. This condition tends to occur on the hands. Patients with Pyoderma gangrenosum may also have involvement of other organ systems that manifest as sterile abscesses.

Healing tends to parallel the activity of the underlying inflammatory bowel disease and permanent scarring is relatively common.

Louis A. Brunsting and his coworkers first described Pyoderma gangrenosum in 1930.

Diseases that are associated with Pyoderma gangrenosum are ulcerative colitis, Crohn's disease, diverticulitis, intestinal polyps, chronic hepatitis, cirrhosis of the liver, sclerosing cholangitis, rheumatoid arthritis, ankylosing spondylitis, systemic lupus erythematosus, Wegner's granulomatosis, Behçet's disease, leukemia, lymphoma, myeloproliferative

74

disorders, carcinoma of breast, lung, colon, or prostate and AIDS.

Pyoderma gangrenosum is seen in about 1 per 100,000 people each year. Death from the disease is rare, it but may occur due to an associated disease or as the result of therapy. Pain is a usual complaint of patients and may require narcotics. There is no apparent racial predilection but it does affect both sexes and there appears to be a slight female predominance.

All ages may be affected, but it is seen predominantly in the fourth and fifth decades. Children may be affected but account for only 3 - 4% of the total cases.

Treatment is usually non-surgical as surgical treatment, known as debridement, may actually cause an increase in the size of the lesions, also called a pathergic reaction. Skin grafting is only performed when the disease is inactive. Treatment is usually successful by arresting the process, but complete healing may take months. If left untreated the ulcers may continue to enlarge, persist unchanged and may not heal.

Often conventional antibiotics are prescribed prior to making the correct diagnosis. These may be continued if bacteria are cultured in the wound causing a secondary infection, but they are not helpful for uncomplicated Pyoderma gangrenosum. Small ulcers are best treated with topical steroid creams, Intralesional steroid injections, special dressings such as silver sulphadiazine cream or hydrocolloids, oral anti-inflammatory antibiotics such as dapsone or minocycline. If tolerated, careful compression bandaging is used for swollen legs.

More severe disease requires immunosuppressive therapy such as oral steroids such as Cyclosporin, which is very expensive, Cyclophosphamide and Methotrexate. These may be required for several months in high dose

75

and there may be severe side effects. See the Medication Index for a list of the side effects for these medications.

Management of Pyoderma gangrenosum continues to be a therapeutic challenge, both because the low incidence of the disease makes it difficult to conduct large-scale randomized studies and because pathogenic mechanisms are not yet well defined. The selection of drugs and dosing schedules is therefore mainly guided by clinical experience.

Systemic effects on the Joints

Sacroiliac

The sacroiliac joint connects the sacrum, which is the triangular or wedged shape bone at the bottom of the spine, with the pelvis, known as the iliac bone. Its purpose is to transmit all the forces of the upper body to the pelvis and legs. There is not a lot of motion in the joint and it is very strong. The wedge shape of the sacrum contributes to the stability of the joint.

In young people, the joint surfaces are rather smooth. As years progress, the surfaces begin to roughen producing friction and additional stability at the joint. The rough surfaces within the joint are reciprocal to the other side of the joint producing joint continuity. Some evidence suggests that the sacral cartilage may transition to fibro-cartilage later in life.

It is not clearly understood why this joint sometimes becomes painful, although some believe it is due to a limitation in its normal motion patterns. It typically results in pain on one side very low in the back or in the buttocks, and is more common in young or middle age women.

Conservative treatment for sacroiliac joint dysfunction generally centers on trying to restore motion in the joint, and can include physical therapy, Chiropractic or osteopathic manipulation or Sacroiliac joint injections. Surgery for fusing the joint is generally not recommended.

Ankylosing spondylitis

Ankylosing spondylitis is a member of the family of diseases that attack the spine called Spondylarthropathies. These diseases also include Reiter's syndrome, some cases of psoriatic arthritis and the arthritis of Inflammatory Bowel Disease.

Ankylosing spondylitis causes arthritis of the spine and sacroiliac joints. It can cause inflammation of the eyes, lungs, and heart valves and varies from intermittent episodes of back pain that occur throughout life to a severe chronic disease that attacks the spine, peripheral joints and other body organs. Severe cases of Ankylosing spondylitis may result in severe joint and back stiffness, loss of motion and deformity as life progresses.

As the spine becomes more rigid, multiple small stress fractures may develop. Since gravity tends to tip the body forward, the patient may develop a flexed forward posture. The same process can develop in the neck and result in a chin on chest deformity. If the deformity becomes severe the spine may be surgically realigned, although this is a major surgical procedure with significant risk of neurological injury.

Generally, treatment for Ankylosing spondylitis is conservative and the symptoms can be managed with non-steroidal anti-inflammatory drugs (NSAID's) and physical therapy exercises that concentrate on maintaining motion in the lumbar spine and hips. Continuing care is critical. This disease is a lifelong problem and those people who fail to continue treatment permanent posture and mobility losses occur.

Indomethacin is most effective, while Dulfasalazine may benefit those with more severe involvement. Peripheral joint arthritis may respond to Methotrexate.

Rehabilitation therapies are essential. Proper sleep and walking positions, coupled with abdominal and back exercises, help maintain posture. Exercises help maintain joint flexibility. Breathing exercises enhance lung capacity, and swimming provides aerobic exercise. Even with optimal treatment, some people will develop an ankylosed or stiff spine, but they will remain functional if this fusion occurs in an upright position.

Some related diseases and conditions for Ankylosing spondylitis are amyloidosis, arthritis, costochondritis and tietze syndrome, Crohn's disease, heel spurs, psoriatic arthritis, reactive arthritis, SAPHO syndrome, ulcerative colitis. Some related medical procedures and test are arthrocentesis, known as joint aspiration, a total hip or a total knee replacement.

The cause of the disease is not known, but almost all of the Spondylarthropathies patients share a common genetic marker, called HLA-B27. In some cases, the disease occurs in these predisposed people after exposure to bowel or urinary tract infections.

Delayed diagnosis is common because symptoms are often attributed to more common back problems. A dramatic loss of flexibility in the lumbar spine is an early sign of the disease. Although most symptoms begin in the lumbar and sacroiliac areas, they may involve the neck and upper back as well. Arthritis may also occur in the shoulder, hips and feet. Some patients have eye inflammation, and more severe cases must be observed for heart valve involvement.

Descriptions of Ligament Functions

Ventral Sacroiliac Ligament (VSL)

The ventral sacroiliac ligament is the anterior thickening of the sacroiliac joint capsule. The superior portion of the ligament is a caudal extension of the iliolumbar ligaments and is significantly thicker than that of the inferior portion of the ligament. Towards the inferior portion of the joint, the VSL begins to taper as it approaches the upper margin of the iliosciatic notch. The thickness of the anterior joint capsule is no more than 2 mm in thickness, being the smallest of the sacroiliac ligaments. This ligamentous structure receives a considerable amount of support from the symphasis pubis and the pelvic ring. When symphasis disruption produces instability of 25 mm, there is great potential for VSL disruption (Jaovisidha et al., 1996). The function of this ligament is to oppose vertical translation and joint distraction (Jaovisidha et al., 1996).

Sacroiliac Ligament (DSL).

The dorsal sacroiliac ligament effectively attaches the posterior superior iliac spine to the sacrum. Directly caudal to the posterior superior iliac spine this ligament is covered by the fascia of the gluteus maximus muscle. It is so stiff that it can easily be confused with a bony prominence during palpation (Vleeming et al., 1996). The DSL prevents excessive contranutation (Vleeming et al., 1996). The dorsal sacroiliac ligament is continuous with the sacrotuberous ligament.

Interosseous Sacroiliac Ligament

79

The Interosseous sacroiliac ligament of the sacroiliac joint is the thickest and strongest ligament of the joint. It is the largest syndesmosis in the body and dwarfs the relative size of the auricular surfaces (Harrison, Harrison, & Troyanovich, 1997) The axial portion of the joint is where the Interosseous sacroiliac ligament lies, adjoining the median, intermediate, and lateral sacral crests to the tuberosity and posterior superior iliac spine of the ilium. This ligament is thought to strongly resist joint separation as well as vertical and anteroposterior translations (Willard, 1995).

Sacrotuberous Ligament

This ligament is thought to be a specialization of the posteroinferior aspect of the joint capsule (Willard, 1995). The lateral band of this ligament stretches from the PSIS to the ischial tuberosity of the os coxa. The medial band attaches the coccygeal vertebrae with the ischial tuberosity. Lastly, the superior band connects the PSIS with the coccygeal vertebrae with an interdigitation of the Interosseous sacroiliac ligament at the sacroiliac joint. This ligament has a very large lever arm at the joint, restricting the amount of nutation that occurs at the sacroiliac joint (Vleeming, Van Wingerden, Snijders, Stoeckart, & Stijnen, 1989).

Sacrosipinous Ligament

The sacrospinous ligament is a specialization of the anteroinferior joint capsule (Willard, 1995). The triangular-shaped ligament projects from the inferior joint capsule and inferior portion of the coccygeal vertebrae to the ischial spine. This ligament also restricts nutation of the sacrum (Harrison, Harrison, & Troyanovich, 1997).

80

Ilioulumbar Ligaments

The iliolumbar ligament stretches from the transverse processes of the 4th & 5th lumbar vertebrae to the iliac crest and Interosseous sacroiliac ligament on the ipsilateral side. The major function of this ligament is to restrict lateral flexion of the lumbar base relative to the Ilium (Harrison, Harrison, & Troyanovich, 1997). It is also thought to prevent translation of the sacrum out of the pelvic girdle (Willard, 1995).

Systemic effects on the Bones

Osteoporosis or Bone Thinning

Bone Types

The human skeleton comprises two different forms of bone. Cortical, or compact bone, accounts for about 80% of the total skeletal mass and is located primarily in the peripheral skeleton, and Trabecular, or spongy bone, constitutes some 70% of the axial or central skeleton, and is resembles a honeycomb of vertical and horizontal bars called trabeculae. It is within this region that human red marrow is almost exclusively located.

Because of these differences, the surface-to-volume ratio is much higher in trabecular bone than cortical bone. Accordingly bone remodeling has a greater effect on trabecular bone. Thus bone remodeling; the process which replaces old bone with new has an annual turnover rate of about 25% in trabecular and 2 - 3% in cortical bone.

Your bones and your skeleton is not merely alive, it is a dynamic 24-hour a day, synergistic factory working together with other systems in your body to keep you healthy. Your bones are made of calcium and other minerals. With the onset of osteoporosis, one of the leading causes of disability in America today, the bones become less dense and more porous rendering them more susceptible to breaking.

Understanding Your Bones

Bones are not static structures but living tissue constantly reformed by remodeling. Every day old bone is removed and replaced with new bone tissue. When more bone is broken down than is replaced this is called demineralization. This causes the bones to weaken and when the structure loses sufficient density, you face eminent danger of a fracture.

Bones continue to increase their density and calcium content until you reach your mid 30s, at which point you probably have attained your peak bone mass. Afterward you may either maintain this mass or begin to lose calcium yearly, but once this process starts, you rarely can increase bone density. The loss of bone density can increase at menopause, when your body ceases producing estrogen which is required to improve bone strength.

When some medications are used for a long period it can cause bone density to diminish.

Stopping Calcium Loss

Eating a diet rich in nutrients that help your bones stay strong is the first step in stopping or slowing the process of osteoporosis. Calcium, magnesium, vitamin D, phosphorus, soy-based foods and fluoride compose the major nutrients that strengthen bone.

Ninety eight percent of your body's calcium resides in your bones. The rest circulates in the blood, taking part in metabolic functions of the body. Because the body cannot manufacture calcium, you must eat calcium in your daily diet to replace the amounts that are constantly lost. When the diet lacks sufficient calcium to replace the amount that is excreted, the body begins to break down bone for the calcium necessary for life-preserving metabolic processes.

Calcium in the diet can generally slow calcium loss from bones, but it usually doesn't replace calcium already gone. Absorbing calcium from your digestive tract requires the presence of vitamin D. As the body ages, the body's ability to produce vitamin D gradually diminishes. Your diet can make up the difference.

Risk factors for Osteoporosis

For women, smoking places you at risk for osteoporosis by lowering your natural estrogen. It does this in three ways. First, smoking during your reproductive years makes your ovaries less efficient in their function of estrogen production. Next, smoking causes menopause to occur about two years earlier than in non-smokers. Lastly, if you chose hormone replacement therapy, HRT for short, for estrogen replacement after menopause, smoking may lower your estrogen level by decreasing your body's ability to use the estrogen you are replacing. Choosing not to smoke is a big step in protecting your bones as well as your general health.

According to the National Osteoporosis Foundation, consuming large amounts of caffeine is thought to increase the calcium excreted in the urine. In addition, high levels of protein and sodium in the diet are also believed to increase calcium excretion. Although more studies of protein and sodium are needed to precisely determine how these substances influence calcium loss you should limit the caffeine, protein and salt you take in.

In addition to a reduction in caffeine, protein and salt, it is believed that the diuretic action of alcohol and caffeine speed skeletal calcium loss and that alcohol may interfere with intestinal absorption of calcium.

Your risk for developing osteoporosis is largely determined by heredity but those things you can control such as a bone-friendly diet, proper nutrition, exercise, smoking, alcohol use and your estrogen level all play an important part as well.

Reducing the risk of Osteoporosis

Along with a bone-friendly diet, proper nutrition, not smoking and limited alcohol use, you should have an exercise program designed to preserve bone. Weight-bearing exercise which includes weight lifting, walking, jogging and jumping rope, places stress on the bones which in turn strengthens bone density and wards off osteoporosis.

Exercise possesses many benefits for preserving bone. Among these benefits, exercise can help you retain the balance necessary to resist falls and strengthen the muscles that keep you erect. Studies performed on women of all ages found that by doing strength training exercises two times a week for a year, without use of estrogen or HRT, women, on average, added three pounds of muscle and lost three pounds of fat. They were also 75% stronger with improved balance and bone density.

Although strength training can be performed by anyone at any age, it is recommended that if you have an unstable medical condition or if you have recently undergone surgery, wait until you recover and speak with your doctor before beginning an exercise program.

84

If you have not exercised in a long time, consult with your doctor and someone knowledgeable in sports medicine before beginning any exercise program.

Information for this section was provided in part by The National Osteoporosis Foundation, PO Box 96616, Washington DC 20077-7456 and The Osteoporosis and Related Bone Diseases National Resource Center.

Other complications and potential health problems

Constipation

Constipation is the most common gastrointestinal complaint in the United States. Alone, constipation results in approximately 2 million annual visits to the doctor but most people treat themselves without seeking medical help. Currently Americans spend some $725 million on laxatives each year.

Poor diet and lack of exercise are usually the causes of constipation. In most cases constipation is temporary and not serious. At one time or another almost everyone gets constipated. Most people find relief by understanding causes, prevention, and seeking proper treatment. Some other common causes of constipation are not enough fiber in the diet, not enough liquids, medications, irritable bowel syndrome, changes in life or routine such as pregnancy, older age, and travel, abuse of laxatives, ignoring the urge to have a bowel movement, and specific diseases such as multiple sclerosis, Crohn's disease and lupus.

In most cases, following some simple guidelines will help relieve symptoms and prevent recurrence of constipation. Eat a well-balanced, high-fiber diet that includes beans, bran, whole grains, fresh fruits, and vegetables. Drink plenty of liquids. Exercise regularly and set aside time after meals for visits to the toilet. Do not ignore the urge to have a bowel movement. Understand that normal bowel habits vary and whenever a significant or prolonged change in bowel habits occurs, check with a doctor. Most people with mild constipation do not need laxatives but the doctor may recommend laxatives for a limited time for those with chronic constipation.

Gallstones

Gallstones are formed from cholesterol, which makes up only five percent of bile. Cholesterol is not very soluble, so in order to remain suspended in fluid, it must be properly balanced with bile salts. If the liver secretes too much cholesterol into the bile or if the bile becomes stagnant and forms a sludge because of a defect in the mechanisms that cause the gallbladder to empty, or if other factors are present, super saturation can occur. Cholesterol may then form gallstones, which is a condition known as Cholelithiasis. The process is very slow and most often painless. Gallstones can range from a few millimeters to several centimeters in diameter.

About 15% of gallstones are known as pigment stones. They are composed of calcium bilirubinate, or calcified bilirubin, which is the substance formed by the breakdown of hemoglobin in the blood. Pigment stones can be black or brown and often form in the gallbladders of people with hemolytic anemia or cirrhosis. Patients may also have a mixture of pigment and cholesterol gallstones.

At any point stones may obstruct the cystic duct, which leads from the gallbladder to the common bile duct, and cause pain called biliary colic, infection and inflammation known as cholecystitis, or all of these. Approximately 15% of people with stones in the

86

gallbladder also have stones in the common bile duct, known as choledocholithiasis. These stones sometimes pass into the small intestine, but also may lodge in the duct and cause distention, infection, or pancreatitis.

Approximately 80% of people with gallstones never experience any symptoms. Most others remain without symptoms for at least two years after stone formation begins. If symptoms do occur, the chance of developing pain is about 2% per year for the first ten years after stone formation, after which the chance for developing symptoms decreases. On average, symptoms take about eight years to develop. The reason for the decline in incidence after ten years is not known, although some physicians suggest that younger, smaller stones may be more likely to cause symptoms than larger ones.

Kidney Stones

Probably the most painful medical condition that most people ever experience is the passing of a kidney stone.

The pain begins as an ache in the back and side. Then it becomes constant and severe. As the urinary system tries to rid itself of the stone sometimes there is burning during urination, blood in the urine, or a frequent urge to urinate. The pain can be so severe that you may pass out. Nausea and vomiting may occur, and the lower abdomen or flank will be painful if touched. One third of kidney stone patients will be hospitalized.

The economic costs of kidney stones are enormous. In the United States 7 - 10 of every 1,000-hospital admissions are due to kidney stones.

Kidney stones can become stuck in any part of the urinary system and in order to locate a kidney stone, your doctor may perform an x-ray or an ultrasound. These procedures will give a good idea of the stone's size and where it is located. Many patients also receive an intravenous pyelogram, in which a special dye is injected into the patient's vein. The dye eventually collects in the urinary system. Once there the dye produces a white contrast when an x-ray is taken. The dye allows your doctor to precisely locate the stone.

It is very important that the stone, if passed, be saved, so that it can be sent to a laboratory for evaluation. Long-term treatment and prevention plans depend on the type of stone. Between 70 - 80% of stones pass on their own in the urine, usually within 48 hours of the start of the symptoms. To catch a stone, patients are asked to urinate into some type of strainer. All pieces of stone, no matter how small, should be collected and given to the doctor. If one stone is analyzed, more may not be needed, since most people develop just one type of stone.

Although kidney stones are very hard, most of the stones that do not pass out of the body on their own can be eliminated without surgery. A process called lithotripsy, which is derived the Greek word for "stone crushing", breaks the stones into tiny fragments. Lithotripsy also is called extra-corporeal shock wave lithotripsy. This procedure has been used in the United States since 1984. It is performed using a machine called a lithotripter. There are different types of lithotripters, but all focus shock waves from outside the body on the kidney stone. Repeated shock waves will cause the kidney stone to disintegrate into tiny particles and these particles pass easily out of the body in the urine.

The bad news is that those who have had one kidney stone are prone to develop others. Without preventive treatment or changes in lifestyle, patients can develop a new stone within a year or two of the first one. About half of patients do develop a stone again within 5 - 10 years, and 80% do so sometime in their lives. The good news is that there definitely are things you can do to reduce your chances of developing another stone.

One of the most important steps that you can take is to simply get into the life-long habit of drinking a lot of liquid; mainly water. Everyone who has had a kidney stone should drink at least 8 ounces of fluid at each meal, between each meal, before bed, and during the night if awakened to urinate. In other words, you should drink a minimum of 7 and preferably 10 - 12 large glasses of fluid in the course of each day. At least half of these should be glasses of water.

Your fluid intake should be spread out as evenly as possible throughout the day. This keeps the urine from becoming concentrated and reduces the chances that crystals which are the building blocks of kidney stones will form. Since the goal is to produce at least 2 quarts of urine a day, you should drink more fluid in very hot weather to make up for that lost by sweating.

A good way to judge whether you're drinking enough is to watch the color of your urine. If your urine is dark and yellow, drink more. It should be pale, almost watery. Urine has more color in the morning when it is most concentrated, but the rest of the time, the less color the better.

Drinking plenty of fluids also reduces the risk of urinary tract infections which is a major cause of struvite stones. Any infections that do occur should be treated promptly and completely.

Depending on the kind of stone involved and the results of laboratory tests, your doctor may advise you to eat less of certain kinds of foods. For example, patients with calcium oxalate or uric acid stones may need to reduce the amount of meat products and table salt in their diets and increase the amount of fiber. You and your physician may work with a dietitian to develop a diet suited to your particular needs. There are prescription medications that help some patients. Diuretics, such as hydrochlorothiazide, decrease calcium excretion. Potassium citrate binds calcium and helps to remove it safely. Allopurinol, which causes the body to produce less uric acid, is sometimes prescribed for patients with gout. It also reduces their risk of forming uric acid or calcium oxalate stones. Patients taking medications still need to drink at least ten 8-ounce glasses of fluid per day. When cystine stone formation can't be controlled by increased fluid levels alone, penicillamine or tiopronin may be prescribed to make it easier for the body to dissolve cystine. Other specific medications may be prescribed by your doctor.

Pancreatitis

Acute inflammation of the pancreas, known as pancreatitis is a condition that can be life threatening. Pancreatitis can result from a condition called choledocholithiasis. This condition is caused because common duct stones may block the pancreatic duct, which carries digestive enzymes. If a gallstone passes through or lodges in the lower common bile duct, pancreatitis can result. It is sometimes difficult to differentiate between pancreatitis and acute cholecystitis but a correct diagnosis is critical since treatment is very different. Blood tests showing high levels of pancreatic enzymes amylase and lipase can usually indicate the diagnosis of pancreatitis.

A simple urine test is currently being used in providing early evidence of possible pancreatitis in patients who come to the emergency room with severe abdominal pain. Imaging techniques are useful in confirming a diagnosis and Ultrasound is used often. A CT scan, along with a number of laboratory tests, can determine the severity of the condition.

The treatment for pancreatitis is intravenous fluids and painkillers and the patient is not allowed to eat or drink anything. Mild cases usually subside within a week. A Cholecystectomy, which is the removal of the gallbladder, is often then performed.

About 25% of pancreatitis cases are severe. Severity appears to be much higher in people who are obese.

Intestinal Gas

Many Crohn's patients are concerned that they have too much intestinal gas. It can be embarrassing and almost always occurs when it is least expected. It is not uncommon to believe that the digestive tract is malfunctioning because of excessive gas. Fear that a serious ailment is present, although concerning, it is rarely the case. It is important to know that gas in itself is not dangerous. However, its consequences may have social implications due to our inability to control its passage.

Intestinal gas can be extremely painful. The abdomen can become painfully bloated or swollen especially right after eating. Sometimes bloating can be so severe that clothing becomes tight and may no longer fit. Because of its severity intestinal gas sufferers can be overly concerned regarding its seriousness. One thing to remember is that all people have gas in the intestinal tract. The amount of gas varies from person to person.

Intestinal gas is generated from two sources: exogenous/ingested; which is essentially swallowed air; and endogenous gas, which is produced by colonic bacteria. Intestinal gas is composed of various amounts of oxygen, nitrogen, carbon dioxide, hydrogen and methane. Oxygen, nitrogen and carbon dioxide come from swallowed air while hydrogen and methane are produced in the colon by bacteria acting on food residue. Analysis of intestinal gas has shown that about ninety percent is ingested air and only ten percent is actually formed in the intestine.

Although less than one percent of gas is odorous, intestinal bacteria produce several sulphur containing compounds that are the primary odor causing culprits. The human nose can detect hydrogen sulphide in concentrations as low as one-half part per billion.

So in other words, if you slip, we will probably know it!

Gas is released from the intestinal tract via the mouth by belching or the rectum as flatus. A normal individual emits flatus about 12 to 25 times per day. In the normal situation swallowed air remains in the stomach for a period of time. Gas passes out of the stomach in small amounts at regular intervals and passes rapidly through the small intestine by means of normal contractions that are involuntary actions by the body. The gas then enters the colon where it passes more slowly but is eventually released through the anus in small amounts.

In most cases intestinal gas can be quite bothersome. There are three common symptoms of intestinal gas: burping or belching, abdominal bloating or distension, and increased flatus.

Swallowed air may be trapped in the stomach and then be released by burping or belching. Since distension of the intestine initiates a contraction, increased gas passing out of the stomach into the intestine may initiate contractions, which if strong enough, may cause cramps. If air is trapped in the small bowel, or more likely in the colon, then bloating and distension may occur. The distension may stimulate spasmodic contractions that prevent the propulsive movement of the gas and thus cause further build-up of the gas and further distension. Gas passing through the bowel will eventually be passed as flatus and gas produced in the colon is also passed as flatus. This gas is usually foul smelling.

Gum chewing, poor fitting dentures, a chronic post nasal discharge, chronic pain, and anxiety or tension, all cause increased air swallowing. Each of these activities should be avoided. Gulping of food and mashing food down with liquids also increases air ingestion and so should be avoided. Beverages should be taken lukewarm and sipping hot drinks avoided. Foods such as lettuce and cabbage, which cannot be chewed into a small bolus, cause increased air to be swallowed and should be used moderately.

The most common source of indigestible carbohydrate is lactose. Lactose is found in such dairy products as milk and milk-based cheese products. Only very small amounts of lactose are found in cream-based and aged cheeses. If you are lactose intolerant commercial products are available to aid the digestion of lactose.

The next most common source of gas is beans. Beans contain the complex carbohydrate raffinose and stachyose which cannot be absorbed by the human intestine. Besides beans and lactose many other fruits and vegetables are gas producers. Because not everyone reacts the same to these foods, eliminating these foods from the diet simply because they produce gas is not recommended.

Intestinal gas is really more of an annoyance than a serious medical problem but excessive gas accompanied by other symptoms, or gas not relieved by dietary changes, should be investigated by your doctor.

Intestinal tuberculosis

Intestinal tuberculosis, which is a known mycobacterial disease and Crohn's disease exhibit extremely similar symptoms. This similarity has caused confusion when diagnosing the diseases; with one disease often being misdiagnosed as the other. In areas of the world where tuberculosis is more prevalent, such as Asia, Crohn's disease is rare, and often mistaken for tuberculosis. In others area, mostly North America and Europe, Crohn's disease is often the diagnosis of choice. This choice is based primarily upon the ability to culture mycobacteria from biopsies of the patient as tested by the acid-fast stain test. If acid-fast mycobacteria are found the diagnosis becomes tuberculosis. Otherwise it becomes Crohn's disease.

Confusion between the intestinal tuberculosis and Crohn's disease is because there is a great degree of similarity between treatments of the two diseases. The correct course of treatment for tuberculosis is a lengthy multi-drug regime of antibiotics, which results in improvement of the patient after some weeks. Crohn's disease patients that have been treated with these same drug regimes have also improved greatly. Similarly tuberculosis patients treated with corticosteroids such as Prednisone experienced a remission of symptoms for periods of up to two months. Unfortunately the disease invariably returns, and its symptoms are exacerbated after this initial remission.

The most important criteria for diagnosing intestinal tuberculosis instead of Crohn's disease is the presence of acid-fast bacilli which is bacteria that become visible when tested by Ziehil-Neelsen acid-fast staining test.

Intestinal tuberculosis comes in two forms: Bacillary and Spheroplast. The spheroplast form is not detectable by the acid-fast stain test. The bacillary form of intestinal tuberculosis is readily detectable by the acid-fast test.

It is theorized that the spheroplast form of mycobacterium paratuberculosis causes Crohn's disease. It is not detectable by the acid-fast stain test.

Amebiasis

Amebiasis is an intestinal infection caused by a microscopic parasite known as Entamoeba histolytica. This parasite produces cysts, called eggs, which are passed from the body in the stool. Anyone can get amebiasis but it occurs more often in people arriving from tropical or subtropical areas, individuals in institutions for the developmentally disabled and homosexual males. Occasionally, amebiasis is misinterpreted to be ulcerative colitis or Crohn's disease.

Most people get amebiasis by eating or drinking contaminated food or water but it can also be spread by oral-anal contact. Oral-anal contact usually occurs when someone with the parasite touches something and another person touches the object or eats the contaminated food. The eggs are swallowed and the infection occurs. People are infectious as long as the eggs are contained in the stool.

Symptoms may be mild, severe or there may be no symptoms at all. Fortunately, most infected people do not become seriously ill. The symptoms of Amebiasis include diarrhea, possibly containing blood, nausea, weight loss, abdominal tenderness, cramps and occasional fever. The symptoms usually start 2 to 4 weeks after infection, but symptoms may not show up for months.

Rarely the parasite will invade the body beyond the intestines and cause a more serious infection, such as a

95

liver abscess. In even more remote cases the parasite may invade the lung, brain, or perforate the colon causing death.

Diagnosis is done by examining a stool sample under a microscope for the presence of the parasite or its eggs. Occasionally, several stool samples must be obtained because the number of eggs found in the stool changes from day to day.

Practicing common sense personal hygiene and developing good hand-washing habits after going to the bathroom or changing diapers is the most effective way to prevent infection. Another excellent prevention measure is to always wash your hands prior to preparing meals.

If household members develop symptoms they should be tested for amebiasis. Food-handlers who are infected should not work until after treatment is finished. Generally, however; it is not necessary to for an infected person to stay home from work or school. Casual contact at work or school is unlikely to cause transmission of the disease, provided that infected and non-infected persons carefully wash their hands after using the toilet.

Your doctor, to treat amebiasis can prescribe specific antibiotics. There are no over-the-counter medications that will cure this infection and once a person is treated, they will no longer carry the parasite in the intestinal tract and are not likely to become ill with amebiasis again.

Anemia

Anemia occurs when the concentration of the red blood cells falls below normal. Red blood cells are essential for delivering oxygen from the lungs to the body's tissue. Patients with Crohn's disease and ulcerative are especially susceptible to anemia because bleeding in the gastrointestinal tract are very common.

Good nutrition is a requirement for adequate red blood cell production and prevention of nutrition-related anemia. Avoidance of nutrition-related anemia depends on adequate dietary intake of iron, vitamin B12, and folate as well as the full complement of other essential nutrients. Folate deficiency anemia usually occurs among women late in the course of pregnancy, small or premature infants, and among alcoholics.

Since Crohn's patients consume little if any red meat or usually have a restricted diet, someone with Crohn's should seek out and take supplemental sources of vitamin B12.

Blood Clots

Blood clots are formed by a cluster of blood cells and fibrin strands that may form in one of the heart's chambers or in a blood vessel that has been injured. The process of forming a blood clot is known as coagulation, which is the blood's normal tendency to plug an injury to prevent further bleeding.

A blood clots name usually refers to the area of the body where the clot occurs. Some examples are pulmonary embolism, which is a blood clot in one of the arteries of the heart. Mesenteric venous thrombosis is a blood clot in the mesenteric veins, which are either of two veins draining the intestine, and retinal vein occlusion refers to a blood clot in a vein of the eye.

Blood clotting is a natural bodily function that regularly occurs as part of the normal healing process. Unfortunately, blood clots sometimes form even when a person has not been wounded in any way. Although most blood clots tend to dissolve on their own and be reabsorbed by the body with no long-term problems,

97

there are four situations in which blood clots can cause life-threatening emergencies.

Arterial Blood Clots

Blood clots that form in an artery, known as a thrombus, could block the flow of blood in the heart and could trigger a heart attack. The arteries most concerning to cause a heart attack are blockage of the coronary arteries. These arteries are located on the surface of the heart.

Another blockage involving arteries of the heart are pulmonary arteries. The pulmonary artery travels from the heart to the lungs and blockage in this artery is called a pulmonary embolism. A pulmonary embolism may result in damage to the lung and can cause death.

When the carotid arteries, which are arteries that lead to the brain, become blocked, this blockage could trigger a stroke or a mini-stroke, known as a transient ischemic attack. A stroke can lead to mild or severe disability, brain damage, and in some instances, death.

The fourth situation that could cause life threatening emergencies is when a piece of a blood clot breaks off in one of the heart's chambers and then travels through the bloodstream. This is known as an embolus.

The blood clot may lodge in an organ or an artery and will either severely diminish or cut off the blood supply from that point. This is called an embolism. An embolism can cause pain known as claudication, a lack of color in the blocked area, weakness in the limb, and if left untreated will cause an infection or tissue death.

Embolisms can be life threatening and emergency treatment is usually necessary.

Venous Blood Clots

A blood clot that forms in the veins is known as a venous blood clot or a peripheral venous disorder.

There are a number of peripheral venous disorders such as a thrombophlebitis whereby an obstructing blood clot form and causes the surrounding vein to become inflamed. This condition is known as phlebitis. If the blood clot formed in a superficial vein near the surface of the skin, it is called superficial vein thrombosis. If the blood clot formed in a deeper vein, it is called deep vein thrombosis.

Another peripheral venous disorder is varicose veins. These are caused when a blood clot damages the valves within a vein and the leaky or damaged valves cause the blood to pool in the legs, resulting in swollen, varicose veins.

The valves are responsible for keeping blood flowing smoothly and in the proper direction, which is particularly important when the veins are counteracting the effects of gravity to bring oxygen-poor blood from the legs to the heart. The valves close between heartbeats to keep blood from flowing backward in the wrong direction known as regurgitation.

Thrombotic thrombocytopenic purpura (TTP) is a condition in which a lack of platelets can lead to the formation of small blood clots throughout the body. Left untreated, TTP can cause widespread damage to many organs throughout the body.

Causes of Blood Clots

Some underlying conditions that could contribute to the formation of blood clots include trauma to a blood vessel due to an accident or a medical procedure, heart attack, stroke, heart disease, congestive heart failure, infection, auto immune disorders, bleeding disorders, Crohn's disease, ulcerative colitis, certain cancers,

99

family history of varicose veins or other vascular conditions, pregnancy, hypertension commonly known as high blood pressure, thrombocythemia, and atrial fibrillation.

Atrial fibrillation is also called AF or A Fib, is the most common abnormal heart rhythm. AF is a very fast, uncontrolled heart rhythm caused when the upper chambers of the heart, the atria, quiver instead of beating. During AF, the upper chambers of the heart beat between 350 and 600 times per minute. Normal heart rhythm is between 60 and 80 beats per minute. Because the pumping function of the upper chambers isn't working properly, the blood is not completely emptied from the heart's chambers, causing it to pool and sometimes clot.

In about 5% of patients with AF, clotted blood dislodges from the atria and results in a stroke. The American Heart Association estimates that in the U.S., AF is responsible for over 70,000 strokes each year.

There are also a number of risk factors that can increase the chances of developing a blood clot. These risk factors include smoking, obesity of more than 20 pounds over the individual's ideal weight, prolonged lack of exercise, oral contraceptive use, advanced age, genetic factors such as inheriting a tendency to develop deep vein thrombosis and sitting in one position for a prolonged period of time.

Symptoms of Blood Clots

The symptoms of a blood clot depend on where the blood clot is located in the body.

A blood clot in a lung may cause sharp chest pain, tachycardia, which is a rapid heart rate, hemoptysis, which is blood-tinged coughing, shortness of breath, or a low-grade fever.

A blood clot that forms in the artery of the arm or leg could cause sudden pain, swelling and slight blue coloration. If the blood clot forms in a vein, it could cause swelling and tenderness.

Blood clots in the brain are very serious. These can lead to visual disturbances, weakness, seizure, speech impairment, stroke or mini stroke.

When bloods clot form in the heart there will be chest pain and left untreated they could lead to a heart attack. Blood clots that form in the heart can also travel to any organ or artery in the body and cause symptoms where the blood clot lodges.

A blood clot in the abdomen will usually cause severe abdominal pain, vomiting and/or diarrhea.

Diagnosing Blood Clots

Diagnosis of a blood clot begins with a complete physical examination and a complete family and personal medical history.

Once a blood clot is suspected, a number of tests can be used to confirm the diagnosis. These tests include:

Doppler ultrasound, which is an imaging technology that uses sound and/or motion waves to produce visual images of the shape and outline of various blood vessels and organs in the body, as well as any obstructions to blood flow.

CT Scan with the use of a special dye or contrast medium being injected prior to imaging.

An MRI or a Magnetic Resonance Angiogram (MRA) is also done after the injection of a dye to view blood flow through the coronary arteries or carotid arteries.

Venograms may be ordered to assess a blood clot in a vein. This diagnostic test involves the use of a dye that is injected into the vein of the affected area prior to the x-ray. The resulting film clearly reveals the shape, size and composition of the vein, as well as any obstructions to blood flow.

Treatments for Blood Clots

The treatments for a blood clot depend on whether the clot has formed in a vein or an artery. If it has formed in an artery and has caused a heart attack or stroke, then thrombolytic medications or clot busters may be used to dissolve the blood clot. These medications are administered to carefully selected patients according to a rigid protocol. To be effective, they must be given within three hours of the heart attack or stroke.

More invasive procedures, such as a catheter directed thrombolysis may be used. In this procedure, the doctor inserts a catheter that delivers thrombolytic enzymes directly to the blood clot. This allows for a higher concentration of the enzymes to be used with fewer side effects than when they are given intravenously. Both types of thrombolytic treatments are then followed by treatment with anticoagulants to prevent additional blood clots from forming.

If a blood clot forms in a vein, there is some risk that a pulmonary embolism will develop. To prevent a pulmonary embolism, blood clots can usually be treated with a combination of heat, painkilling medications, anticoagulants, elevation and bandaging of the affected area to reduce swelling.

In extreme situations, surgery may be required to remove a clot from the heart before it breaks apart starts to travel to other parts of the body. One surgical method uses a vena caval filter, in which a small metallic screening device is placed directly into the heart via a vein known as the inferior vena cava, to trap blood clots before they travel.

Due to the invasiveness of this procedure, this method is only used when the patient cannot tolerate and/or does not respond to other forms of thrombolytic therapy.

Each patient's treatment will depend on the location of the clot, the size of the clot and the patient's general health.

Prevention of Blood Clots

Prevention plans and strategies are particularly important to people who are prone to blood clots. The best strategy for preventing blood clots is to exercise regularly. Regular exercise can be one of the best methods of preventing blood clots from forming because it promotes good circulation.

Maintaining a healthy weight and not smoking are equally important in preventing blood clots. For those confined to a bed or chair, regular movement and stretching is vital. You should also avoid sitting with crossed legs and wearing tight garments below the waist.

Doctors may also prescribe antiplatelets to help prevent blood clots.

Whenever a patient undergoes a surgical procedure, there is the possibility of blood clot formation during the surgery or recovery period. To reduce the risk of blood clots, anticoagulants may be prescribed especially after orthopedic procedures on the hip or knee. Performing calf and leg exercises before surgery and resuming activity as soon as possible after surgery can be helpful in blood clot prevention.

After surgery, cuffs that inflate intermittently may be wrapped around the patient's legs to improve circulation and reduce the risk of blood clots.

If you are scheduled for a surgical procedure, you should discuss the risk factors with your doctor.

Heartburn / Indigestion and other related conditions

In the United States, almost 50% of the population experience heartburn at least once a month and 7% have it daily. Heartburn is even more common during pregnancy, with about 1 in 4 women reporting it daily at some point during their pregnancy. Statistics on acid indigestion are difficult to find because the definition is vague, but it's probably almost as common as heartburn.

Heartburn

Heartburn is a burning feeling in the middle of your chest caused by acid leaking upwards from the stomach into the esophagus at the stomach/esophagus junction. This condition is known as Esophagitis.

Normally, the muscular esophagus acts like a one-way valve allowing food to enter your stomach after swallowing, but not letting anything go back up. When your esophagus is too loose where it connects to the stomach, strong stomach acid seeps back through the opening and causes heartburn.

Because your esophagus doesn't have a protective lining like the stomach, the esophagus can be burned by the acid, causing pain and sometimes damage. This damage can be permanent and can eventually lead to cancer of the esophagus. Heartburn can also cause nighttime cough, wheezing, and in some cases difficulty swallowing food due to scarring of the esophagus.

To prevent stomach acid from splashing back up into the esophagus and causing heartburn, you must tighten the loose esophagus where it meets the stomach. Avoiding certain foods and activities can stop the problem in many cases. But for those with a Hiatal hernia, which is a bulging of the stomach partly into the chest cavity, overweight people, and pregnant women, it may not be able to improve the reflux of acid into the esophagus/stomach junction. In those cases, gravity seems to be the best source for help.

Just staying upright long enough to let food and acid empty out of your stomach in mist cases can stop the problem. To prevent heartburn never lay down after a meal, allow 2-3 hours between eating and bed time and try propping up the head of your bed 2 or 3 inches with books or blocks under the legs of the frame. It's hard for stomach acid to go uphill into your esophagus.

There are several foods and activities that loosen the esophagus or promote heartburn in other ways. Foods to avoid are alcohol, peppermint/spearmint, chocolate, all caffeinated drinks such as coffee, tea and many soft drinks, spicy and fatty foods. Activities to avoid are smoking, eating before bed, and lying down after a meal and tight waisted clothing.

Along with the foods and activities listed above, many prescription medications cause heartburn. If you take certain high blood pressure medications, tranquilizer or anti-depressants, or female hormones, check with your doctor if you experience heartburn

Acid Indigestion

Acid indigestion is a similar burning discomfort, but the sensation is in the pit of your stomach. Acid indigestion can be caused by acid irritating the stomach lining or duodenum. Acid indigestion is believed to happen not just because of too much acid, but also because of too little protection from the mucus lining the stomach. Acid indigestion can burn so deeply into your stomach or duodenum that a canker sore-like crater forms. This is known as Peptic ulcer disease, or a Peptic ulcer. A Peptic ulcer usually needs to be treated by a physician.

Fortunately, you can prevent Heartburn, Acid indigestion and Peptic ulcers by following a few simple steps and using newly available over the counter medicines to stop problems in their early stages.

To prevent acid indigestion, you need to protect the stomach lining and avoid activities that increase stomach acid. To help maintain the protective layer of the stomach, don't take Aspirin, Ibuprofen, or other NSAID's of this type as they can directly damage your protective stomach lining. Acetaminophen products will not cause such damage. Don't smoke or use any tobacco products because nicotine and other substances found in tobacco both weaken the stomach's protective layer and increase acid production.

To stop your stomach from producing extra acid, avoid all coffee, all caffeinated products, chocolate, carbonated drinks, citrus fruits and juices, alcohol, spicy foods and milk (Surprise! Milk may actually aggravate your acid indigestion, not soothe it.)

Treatment of Heartburn and Acid Indigestion

Self-treatment of heartburn and acid indigestion is easier and more effective than ever before, thanks to super-potency antacids and the new H_2 blockers. But you can not lose site of the fact that this is one of the few self-treatment health conditions that can actually progress to a potentially life-threatening situation. If you experience any of the following conditions, you should contact your doctor immediately: Black stools, a frequent nighttime cough, awaken at night with a choking sensation or foul taste in the back of the throat, or have difficulty swallowing or a sensation that food gets stuck half way down.

It's important to know when your condition has gone beyond the self-treatment stage.

Heartburn and acid indigestion should cause fairly mild pain. If the discomfort is severe enough to prevent normal functioning at work, home, or school, or is not completely and consistently relieved by the medications and other measures discussed in this section, you should seek prompt evaluation by your doctor.

Diabetic gastroparesis

Diabetic gastroparesis is a condition in which the stomach does not contract. The symptoms for this include vomiting, nausea, heartburn, indigestion, a persistent fullness after meals, and appetite loss.

Gastro esophageal reflux disease

Gastroesophageal reflux disease is a back flow of acid into the canal to the stomach and Erosive esophagitis is severe inflammation of the esophageal canal. This condition, if left untreated, can lead to cancer.

Chapter 6

Diagnosis

Crohn's disease diagnoses techniques are similar to the diagnosis of ulcerative colitis. The difference between the diagnosis techniques are found by studying the nature and location of the specific inflammation. The specific diagnosis of Crohn's is made based on symptoms and the exclusion of other diseases by observation of typical findings with an endoscopy and failure to find evidence of infection.

It is possible to tell the difference between Crohn's disease and ulcerative colitis, however; determining the difference can be difficult. Specifically, there may be some uncertainty whether it is Crohn's disease or ulcerative colitis affecting the colon. This condition is called indeterminate colitis. Occasionally a diagnosis of ulcerative colitis will eventually turn out to be Crohn's disease.

Additional testing to help make the diagnosis may include barium x-rays of the upper and lower gastrointestinal tract. Barium is a chalky material that is visible by x-ray and appears white on x-ray films. These x-rays can be used to define the distribution, nature, and severity of the disease and can show ulceration, swelling, narrowing, and, sometimes, fistulae of the bowel.

Oral Barium X-Ray (Upper GI)

When ingested orally, pictures can be taken of the stomach and the small intestines.

Barium Enema X-Ray (Lower GI)

When barium is administered through the rectum, pictures of the colon and the part of the ileum closest to the colon can be obtained.

In both cases, once the mixture coats the organs, x-rays are taken that reveal their shape and condition. The patient may feel some abdominal cramping when the barium fills the colon, but usually will feel little discomfort after the procedure. Stools may be a whitish color for a few days after the exam.

The night before the test, bowel cleansing, also called bowel prep, is necessary to clear the lower digestive tract. A clean bowel is important, because even a small amount of stool in the colon can hide details and result in an inaccurate exam.

Additional Examinations

Other exams are the flexible sigmoidoscopy, and sometimes a colonoscopy. If inflammation is seen by these techniques, the physician will then attempt to rule out an infectious cause with stool cultures and blood tests. Because Crohn's often mimics other conditions and symptoms may vary widely, the correct diagnosis of Crohn's disease may take some time.

Sigmoidoscopy

A sigmoidoscopy is an examination of the rectum and lower colon, also known as the sigmoid colon. The night before a sigmoidoscopy, the patient usually has a liquid dinner and takes an enema in the early morning.

A light breakfast and a cleansing enema an hour before the test may also be necessary.

To perform a sigmoidoscopy, the doctor uses a long, flexible tube with a light on the end called a sigmoidoscope to view the rectum and lower colon. The patient is not sedated before the exam. First, the doctor examines the rectum with a gloved, lubricated finger. Then, the sigmoidoscope is inserted through the anus into the rectum and lower colon. The procedure may cause a mild sensation of wanting to move the bowels and abdominal pressure. Sometimes the doctor fills the organs with air to get a better view and the air may cause mild cramping.

Colonoscopy

A colonoscopy is more accurate than barium x-rays in detecting small ulcers or small areas of inflammation in the bowel and in assessing the activity and the degree of inflammation. A colonoscopy also allows for small tissue samples to be taken and sent for examination under the microscope to confirm the diagnosis of Crohn's disease.

To perform a colonoscopy, the doctor uses a flexible tube with a light on the end called a colonoscope to view the entire colon. This tube is longer than a sigmoidoscope. The same bowel cleansing used for the barium x-ray is needed to clear the bowel of waste. The patient is lightly sedated before the exam. During the exam, the patient lies on his or her side and the doctor inserts the tube through the anus and rectum into the colon. If an abnormality is seen, the doctor can use the colonoscope to remove a small piece of tissue for examination. The patient may feel gassy and bloated after the procedure.

Digital Rectal Exam

A physical exam may include a digital rectal exam. This is performed with a gloved, lubricated finger to evaluate the tone of the muscle that closes off the anus, known as the anal sphincter. It also is used to detect tenderness, obstruction, or blood. In some cases, blood and thyroid tests may be necessary.

CAT / CT Scans

A computerized axial tomography (CAT or CT) scanning is a computerized x-ray technique that allows imaging of the entire abdomen and pelvis. It can be especially helpful in detecting abscesses.

Other Considerations

The Doctor should consider a diagnosis of Crohn's disease if the patient has a fever, abdominal pain and / or tenderness, diarrhea with or without bleeding, and anal diseases. Laboratory blood tests may show elevated white cell counts and sedimentation rates, both indicating infection or inflammation. Other blood tests may show low red cell counts, known as anemia, low blood proteins, and low body minerals, reflecting loss of these elements due to chronic diarrhea.

Extensive testing usually is reserved for people with severe symptoms, for those with sudden changes in number and consistency of bowel movements or blood in the stool, and for older adults. Because of an increased risk of colorectal cancer in older adults, the doctor may use other tests to rule out a diagnosis of cancer.

WARNING!!!! I have lived with the result of an incorrect diagnosis and improperly performed surgical procedure. Before undergoing any hemorrhoid surgery or any other surgery for any other symptom, make sure that your surgeon is fully aware of, and has properly diagnosed Crohn's disease. <u>**Incorrect diagnosis and improper surgery can cause serious and permanent injury to your body.**</u>

Chapter 7

Crohn's Disease and Women

Women who have Crohn's disease or ulcerative colitis are naturally concerned about the impact that these diseases may have on fertility and pregnancy. This Chapter focuses on women, fertility, gynecology, birth and medications taken during pregnancy.

Pregnancy

Generally, women with Crohn's disease whose disease is inactive have the same ability to conceive as women in the general population who don't have these diseases. Women whose disease is under good control with medical treatment also have no difficulty in becoming pregnant, but a woman who is in poor nutritional condition due to Crohn's disease may find it difficult to become pregnant.

For women whose Crohn's is active, they may experience gynecological complications that reduce their ability to become pregnant. When the illness is very active in the small intestine, the inflammation may interfere with function of the ovaries. Crohn's may also cause pelvic scarring, and abscesses and fistulas to and around the vagina may interfere with intercourse.

When the disease is brought back under control, the woman's ability to conceive is almost always restored.

Studies suggest that women, who have ulcerative colitis, whether active or inactive, have no apparent problems regarding fertility.

Fear of Pregnancy

Many women with Crohn's are afraid to become pregnant for fear of having a complicated pregnancy or an abnormal baby at birth. Most women with Crohn's will be able to conceive and to deliver healthy, full-term babies.

A woman whose illness is under good control or is mildly active should not fear becoming pregnant, Gastroenterologists generally recommend that those who have significantly active disease with abdominal pain and diarrhea should wait to become pregnant until the illness goes into remission or improves significantly.

At least 80% of women with inactive Crohn's will experience a normal full-term delivery. This is comparable to the general population of women who do not have the disease. A flare-up of the disease or temporary worsening of symptoms is not a contraindication to continuing the pregnancy, since it usually can be brought under control with medical therapy.

Women with active Crohn's, especially women who develop the disease during pregnancy, have two to three times' greater chance of a spontaneous abortion or a pre-term birth. The increased risk to the fetus is not due to drug therapy, but to the activity of the disease itself.

Delivery Options

A major concern of women who become pregnant and have had previous surgery for Crohn's such as colectomy, ileostomy, continent ileostomy or ileoanal anastomosis, is whether they can have a normal delivery or must have a Caesarean section.

The good news is that the vast majority of women with Crohn's will be able to have a normal vaginal delivery. Normal delivery is far more preferable to a Caesarean section unless there are obstetrical reasons to perform the latter.

The not so good news is that women with severe perineal disease such as rectovaginal fistulas or abscesses are strongly recommended to undergo Caesarean section.

Ileostomy Complications

During the course of the pregnancy, enlargement of the abdomen may cause some problems with the size and contour of the ileostomy, necessitating a larger appliance. A prolapse, known as slippage, of the ileostomy may occur. This usually is not a problem, since a small protrusion of the ileostomy remains after the prolapse.

As the pregnancy progresses a woman who has undergone ileostomy surgery should avoid wearing a belt, which can increase abdominal pressure and cause further prolapse of the ileostomy.

Occasionally, at the end of the third trimester, the ileostomy may be displaced by the enlarging uterus and may result in a partial obstruction of the small intestine. This may require the induction of labor earlier than the expected date of delivery.

Treatment during Pregnancy

Pregnancy usually proceeds normally in women who have had previous intestinal resection if the Crohn's is inactive. The fetus usually has fared well in cases where

115

surgery is required late in pregnancy for either very severely active Crohn's, toxic mega colon, or for obstruction or perforation of the bowel. If surgery is required earlier in the course of the pregnancy there is a 50% incidence of spontaneous abortion or premature birth.

If at all possible, your doctor should optimize medical therapy to enable you to plan the timing of your pregnancy with remission of your Crohn's. If a flare-up of the disease occurs during pregnancy, you need not fear routine medical therapy as this should not threaten the fetus and should help induce remission.

In short, women who have inactive Crohn's or if the disease is under control with medication can anticipate an uncomplicated pregnancy ending with a full-term, healthy baby.

Medications during Pregnancy

If the disease is inactive, avoidance of all medication is the best treatment. When Crohn's is active, it is generally safe to use sulfasalazine and definitely 5-ASA drugs, as well as corticosteroids.

Antibiotics and immunomodulator medications should be avoided, as there is not enough knowledge about the effects of these drugs on pregnancy. If a woman with severe Crohn's does become pregnant and must continue with immunomodulator therapy, she should be aware that recent data indicate a minimal risk to the fetus.

Because researchers do not yet know enough about the potential side effects of antidiarrheal medications, such as Imodium® and Lomotil®, pregnant women should avoid these medications, especially during the first trimester. If possible, use of narcotic antidiarrheals, such as codeine and deodorized tincture of opium, DTO

116

for short, should be avoided because of concern for addiction of the newborn.

Diet

If possible, women with Crohn's should follow the well-balanced diet that is generally recommended to all pregnant women. However, if a woman with Crohn's is unable to absorb sufficient nutrients from such a diet, her doctor may suggest nutritional supportive therapy. This may include special liquid formulas that supply vital nutrients.

Breastfeeding

Most medications are safe to take during breastfeeding, but there are a few that can be dangerous for your baby. To be sure that you avoid any potential problems with medications, let your doctor and your baby's pediatrician know that you are breastfeeding. Make sure to get approval for all medications, including non-prescription drugs and always take the medication just after you nurse rather than just before.

Many parents are concerned that breastfeeding has to stop if the mother suffers a relapse. During most illnesses such as a cold, the flu, bacterial infections, surgical conditions, and even during a relapse, breastfeeding can and should continue. Both the mother and baby benefit if breastfeeding continues without interruption.

If you are breastfeeding, by the time you show symptoms of an illness, your baby has already been exposed to it so the best thing to do is to keep breastfeeding. Since you have already started to produce antibodies, through your milk you will protect your baby from getting infected. If you stop breastfeeding when cold or flu symptoms appear, you actually reduce your baby's protection and increase the chance of the baby getting sick. You cannot transmit Crohn's disease or ulcerative colitis to your baby by breastfeeding.

If you are unable to breastfeed your infant while you are ill, keep up your milk supply by expressing milk for your baby either by hand or using a pump. The milk can then be fed to the baby by bottle.

Even with more serious illnesses, such as a breast abscess, surgery, or severe infections caused by a relapse, you usually only need to stop breastfeeding for a short period. There are only a few infectious diseases that mothers have that can be transmitted through human milk to the baby. These include HIV, hepatitis, and untreated tuberculosis.

If you are diagnosed with HIV, it is highly recommended that you do not breastfeed your child. Mothers with tuberculosis should not breastfeed until appropriate treatment has been started. Mothers with hepatitis B can breastfeed their infants if the infant receives the hepatitis B vaccine in the first few days after birth. There is no evidence that hepatitis C is transmitted by breastfeeding and mothers with chronic hepatitis C are often advised that they can breastfeed their infants. If you have chronic hepatitis C, this option should be discussed with your doctor.

Other types of infections need to be evaluated by your doctor and the baby's pediatrician, but nearly all will be found to be safe for breastfeeding.

Newborn Baby Complications

Necrotizing enterocolitis

Necrotizing enterocolitis is a serious bacterial infection in the intestine, primarily of sick or premature newborn infants. Necrotizing enterocolitis most commonly affects the lower portion of the small intestine and it is less common in the colon and upper small bowel. It can cause ulceration, perforations of the bowel, and can progress to necrosis of intestinal tissue and septicemia, known as blood poisoning, which is a life threatening condition in infants.

Simply put, necrotizing enterocolitis shows the exact same symptoms as Crohn's disease does in adults and as with Crohn's the cause of necrotizing enterocolitis is not clear.

Causes and Symptoms

Necrotizing enterocolitis almost always occurs in the first month of life. Infants who require tube feedings may have an increased risk for the disorder. A number of other conditions also make newborns susceptible, including respiratory distress syndrome, congenital heart problems, and episodes of apnea, which is the cessation of breathing. Though the primary risk factor seems to be prematurity. Not only is the undeveloped digestive system less able to protect itself, but premature infants are subjected to many stresses on the body in their attempt to survive.

Early symptoms of necrotizing enterocolitis include an intolerance to formula, distended and tender abdomen, vomiting, and blood both visible or not, in the stool.

One of the earliest signs may also be the need for mechanical support of the infant's breathing. If the infection spreads to the bloodstream, infants may develop lethargy, fluctuations in body temperature, and periodically stop breathing.

Diagnosis

The key to reducing the complications of this disease is early suspicion by your doctor. A series of x-rays of the bowel often reveal the progressive condition, and blood tests will confirm infection.

Treatment

Over two-thirds of infants can be treated without surgery. Aggressive medical therapy starts as soon as the condition is diagnosed or even suspected. Tube feedings directly into the digestive system, referred to as enteral nutrition, are discontinued, and tube feedings into the veins, called parenteral nutrition, are used instead until the condition has resolved. Intravenous fluids are given for several weeks while the bowel heals.

Some infants may be placed on a ventilator to help them breathe and some may receive transfusions of platelets, which will help the blood clot when there is internal bleeding. Antibiotics are usually given intravenously for at least 10 days.

Infants requiring ventilator assistance or transfusion of platelets require frequent evaluations by the doctor. Multiple abdominal x-rays and blood tests to monitor their condition during the illness may also be required.

Sometimes, necrotizing enterocolitis must be treated with surgery. This is often the case when an infant's condition does not improve with medical therapy or there are signs of worsening infection.

The surgical treatment depends on the individual patient's condition. Patients with infection that has caused serious damage to the bowel may have portions of the bowel removed. It is sometimes necessary to create a substitute bowel by making an ostomy into the abdomen through the skin.

Many physicians are avoiding the ostomy and operating to remove diseased bowel and repair the defect at the same time.

Postoperative complications are common, including wound infections and lack of healing, persistent sepsis and bowel necrosis. A serious internal bleeding disorder known as disseminated intravascular coagulation is also common.

Prognosis

Necrotizing enterocolitis is the most common cause of death in newborns undergoing surgery. The average mortality is 30 - 40%. This percentage increases in severe cases.

Early identification and treatment are critical to improving the outcome for infants afflicted with this disease. Aggressive nonsurgical support and careful timing of surgical intervention have improved overall survival, but this condition can be fatal in about one-third of cases. With the resolution of the infection, the bowel may begin functioning within weeks or months. Infants need to be carefully monitored by a physician for years because of possible future complications.

About 10 - 35% of all survivors will eventually develop a stricture that can create an intestinal obstruction, which will require surgery to repair. Infants may also be more susceptible to future bacterial infections in the digestive system and to a delay in growth. Infants with severe cases may also suffer neurological impairment.

The most serious long-term complication associated with necrotizing enterocolitis is short-bowel syndrome. This refers to a condition that can develop when a large amount of bowel must be removed, making the

121

intestines less able to absorb certain nutrients and enzymes.

Infants with short bowel syndrome gradually evolve from tube feedings to oral feedings, and medications are used to control the malabsorption, diarrhea, and other consequences of this condition.

Prevention

In very small or sick premature infants, the risk for necrotizing enterocolitis may be diminished by beginning parenteral nutrition and delaying enteral feedings for several days to weeks.

It has been suggested that breast milk provides substances that may be protective, but there is no evidence that this reduces the risk of infection.

A large multicenter trial showed that steroid drugs given to women in preterm labor might protect their offspring from necrotizing enterocolitis.

Sometimes necrotizing enterocolitis occurs in clusters, or outbreaks, in hospital newborn or neonatal units. Because there is an infectious element to the disorder, infants with necrotizing enterocolitis may be isolated to avoid infecting other infants. Persons caring for these infants must also employ strict measures to prevent spreading the infection.

Information for this section was provided, in part, by Gale Encyclopedia of Medicine. Gale Research, 1999.

For further information on this disease, the following book provides very good information that you can use for your child. "Pediatrics and Genetics: Disturbances in Newborns and Infants." In *The Merck Manual.* Whitehouse Station, NJ, Merck & Co., Inc., 1992.

Gynecological Complications

Ulcerative colitis generally causes few gynecological problems. On the other hand, in those cases where Crohn's disease affects the anal and genital areas and their surrounding tissues, known as the perineum, women may experience numerous gynecological complications. Crohn's disease of the perineum occurs in about 25 percent of all patients.

Menstrual Cycle

Crohn's disease usually does not affect the menstrual cycle, but if active disease causes the body to become debilitated, women may suffer from erratic ovulation and irregular periods. Corticosteroids also may cause irregularities in the menstrual cycle or amenorrhea, which is the absence of periods. When Crohn's is brought back under control, normal menstrual cycles usually resume.

Pelvic Complications

Some women develop a pelvic mass caused by inflammation in the bowel and the surrounding tissues. This condition will improve when the disease is brought back under control.

Fistulas may develop between the intestine and uterus. This was cause chronic inflammation and infection of the endometrium, which is the lining of the uterus; intermittent pelvic pain, and, possibly, low-grade fevers. There also have been cases of fistulas from either the small or large intestine to the vagina. If a vaginal fistula occurs, antibiotics and immunosuppressives may be used to treat the infection. With medication, the fistulas may improve and, on occasion, close. If medication treatment fails, the segment of intestine causing the problem is removed. In some cases, a temporary ileostomy is performed to direct the intestinal contents away from the vagina and allow the fistula to heal.

When a diseased portion of intestine adheres to the fallopian tube and ovary, a tubo-ovarian abscess or a pocket of pus will form. This condition creates a fistula between the intestine and the reproductive organs and the tube and ovary become infected, from which an abscess may form. Some women can be treated with antibiotics while others may require surgical removal of the affected tube and ovary, along with the diseased segment of intestine.

When blisters, sores, or pimples form on the labia, they are actually are tiny fistulas. While some sores heal, others will recur. Antibiotics and immunosuppressive therapy are used in advanced cases. Rarely, medical treatment does not work and the ulcers become very severe. If the condition does not heal or gets worse, the affected portion of the intestine may then have to be surgically removed and an ileostomy created.

Intestinal Surgery and Infertility

After any abdominal operation, adhesions or scar tissue may occur. In women with Crohn's disease, these adhesions may cause blockage, immobility of the fallopian tubes, and ultimately infertility.

In the past, the standard treatment was more abdominal surgery to remove the adhesions. Today, it is possible to bypass the tubes with in-vitro fertilization.

Sexual Intercourse

124

Because severe complications can affect a woman's enjoyment of sex and her ability to have children, her gynecologist and gastroenterologist should work as a team to provide the best treatment possible.

Women and their partners should not hesitate to seek counseling to help them cope with these difficult issues.

Chapter 8

Clinical Depression

A depressed mood and/or general loss of interest that lasts more than two weeks characterize clinical depression. Someone with clinical depression will display a noticeable change from normal functioning and will usually be significantly impaired by its symptoms. Clinical depression can be the result of drug effects, a general medical condition, or the onset of a chronic illness. *Do not confuse clinical depression with normal grief.*

Someone suffering from clinical depression will show many of the following symptoms:

Depressed Mood

A person with a depressed mood will show signs of being sad, cranky or irritable and may display these signs with or without warning. Excessive physical complaints and apathy also define this symptom.

Loss of Interest in or Pleasure from Most Activities

Loss of interest is a symptom may take the form of just "not caring anymore". This may include loss of interest in hobbies or other activities that the patient once enjoyed. An example of this would be where someone who enjoys playing golf suddenly finds excuses not to play. Other activities may be a decreased interest in sex. This lack of interest is referred to as anhedonia.

Indecisiveness or Diminished Ability to Concentrate

This symptom may take the form of being easily distracted or having memory difficulties. Jobs or functions that require concentration may become almost impossible to perform.

Recurrent Thoughts of Death

Thoughts of one's own death are common in depression and should be taken very seriously. These thoughts or feelings can range from a general feeling that others would be better off if the person were dead to making specific suicide plans and preparations. If any of these feelings are displayed, they should always be treated as an emergency and they do require immediate medical attention.

Insomnia

Insomnia or sleeping difficulties can mean difficulty falling asleep, staying asleep, restlessness during the night, or waking up earlier than usual and not being able to fall back to sleep. There are meds available to help treat insomnia.

Hypersomnia, or feeling sleepy and napping all the time, is less common but also occurs.

Fatigue or Loss of Energy

Minor physical activity such as getting dressed may feel like a huge exertion and may take much longer than normal.

Feelings of Worthlessness or Excessive Guilt

Often someone with clinical depression will display these symptoms. Feelings of unrealistic negative self-evaluations, unrealistic self-blame, very low self-esteem or a sense of guilt can reach delusional proportions. If this happens, many other depression symptoms begin to unveil themselves and suicidal tendencies may occur. If any other symptoms occur with any feelings of worthlessness, they should be treated as an emergency and medical attention should be sought out.

Significant Weight Loss or Gain

An example of "significant" weight loss or gain could be gaining or losing over 5% of your body weight in a month, when not dieting or trying to gain weight. Weight gain or loss is usually the result of changes in appetite.

Psychomotor Agitation or Retardation

Psychomotor agitation may appear as pacing, having trouble sitting still, hand wringing, or pulling at skin. Some common examples of psychomotor retardation can include either long pause before answering questions and/or slowed thinking, speaking, and moving.

Types of Depression

Depression is similar to other disorders and diseases because depression comes in different forms or types. If you suspect depression in yourself of someone you know, immediately contact your doctor.

Some of the most common types of depression are addressed and outlined in the *Diagnostic and Statistical Manual of Mental Disorders, Fourth Edition.* Physicians and mental health experts use this publication to classify or describe mental disorders. It is important to note that within each type of depression, there are wide variations in the severity and number of symptoms.

The Wakefield Questionnaire

The Wakefield Questionnaire is presented here to help you become more familiar with the signs and symptoms of depression. Only a professional can diagnose depression, therefore, the Wakefield Questionnaire is by no means intended to replace a visit to your doctor or to a mental health professional. After you complete the statements you should share them with your doctor or mental health professional. Doing this will help to open a dialogue about depression.

The Wakefield Questionnaire contains groups of statements with three established responses. Write these down on a piece of paper and read each group of statements carefully. Mark the answer that best completes each statement as it applies to you. Make sure you choose the statement that describes how you are feeling now, not how you were feeling or how you hope to feel in the future. Complete each statement honestly.

The three responses are:

> No, not at all,
> Yes, sometimes,
> Yes, definitely

The statements are as follows:

I feel miserable and sad.
I find it easy to do the things I used to do.
I get very frightened or panicky feeling for
apparently no reason at all.
I have weeping spells, or feel like it
I still enjoy the things I used to.
I am restless and can't keep still.
I get off to sleep easily without sleeping tablets.
I feel anxious when I go out of the house on my
own.
I have lost interest in things.
I get tired for no reason.
I am more irritable than usual.
I wake early and then sleep badly for the rest of
the night.

Depression can be serious and should be discussed with your doctor. Don't be afraid to bridge the subject even if you don't think or believe you suffer from depression. Having a chronic illness such as Crohn's disease provides the perfect avenue for someone to become depressed and not even know it.

Speak to your doctor or mental health professional candidly about depression and its affects on you.

Antidepressant Medications

The kind of depression that will most likely benefit from treatment with anti-depression medication is more than just general sadness or the blues. Antidepressants are used mostly for serious depressions, but they can also be helpful for some milder depressions. Antidepressants are not stimulants. These medications just eliminate or reduce the symptoms of depression and help the depressed person feel the way they did before they became depressed.

Antidepressants are also used for disorders characterized by anxiety. They block the symptoms of panic, including rapid heartbeat, terror, dizziness, chest pains, nausea, and breathing problems. Antidepressant medication can also be used to treat some phobias.

Some people have one episode of depression and then never experience another, or remain depression free for years. Others have more frequent episodes or very long lasting depressions. These cases may go on for years. As people get older, some find that their depressions become more frequent and severe. An effective way of reducing the frequency and severity of depressions for these people is continuing and on-going treatment with antidepressant medications.

The commonly used antidepressant medications have no known long-term side effects and use may be continued indefinitely. The dosage of antidepressants varies, depending on the type of drug, the person's body chemistry, age, and, sometimes, body weight. Dosages are generally started low and raised gradually over time until the desired effect is reached without the appearance of troublesome side effects. If necessary, the prescribed dosage of the medication may be lowered if side effects become troublesome.

There are a number of antidepressant medications currently available. They differ in their side effects and, to some extent, in their level of effectiveness. Tricyclic antidepressants, which are named for their chemical structure, are more commonly used for treatment of major depressions. Monoamine oxidase inhibitors are often helpful in what is called "atypical" depressions. Atypical depressions cause symptoms like oversleeping, anxiety, panic attacks, and phobias.

131

The last few years have seen the introduction of a number of new antidepressant medications. These new antidepressant medications are called Selective Serotonin Reuptake Inhibitors or "SSRIs for short. The SSRI's that are available at the present time in the United States are fluoxetine (*Prozac*), fluvoxamine (*Luvox*), which has been approved for obsessive-compulsive disorder; paroxetine (*Paxil*) which has been approved for panic disorder; *(Celexa)* which increases the supply of a substance in the brain called serotonin without affecting many of the other chemicals in the brain that influence mood; and sertraline (*Zoloft*).

Although each SSRI is structurally different from each other, all the SSRIs' antidepressant effects are due to their action on one specific neurotransmitter, Serotonin.

The FDA has also approved two other antidepressants that affect the two neurotransmitters Serotonin and Norepinephrine. These antidepressant medications are venlafaxine (Effexor) and nefazodone (Serzone).

All of these newer antidepressants seem to have less bothersome side effects than the older tricyclic antidepressants.

Choosing the correct antidepressant medication

After an examination of the symptoms, your doctor will select the particular antidepressant to prescribe based on the individual patient's symptoms.

When the patient begins taking an antidepressant medication, improvement generally will not begin to show immediately. With most of these medications, it will take from 1 - 3 weeks before changes begin to

132

occur. Some symptoms diminish early in treatment while other symptoms diminish or are eliminated later.

Some patients will respond better to one medication than another. Since there is no certain way of determining beforehand which medication will be effective, the doctor may have to prescribe one, then another until an effective treatment is found.

Side effects of Tricyclics

When taking tricyclic antidepressants, there are a number of possible side effects that vary in severity, depending on the specific medication taken. For example, one tricyclic medication may make people feel drowsy, while another may have an opposite effect, producing feelings of anxiety and restlessness. This large variation in side effects defines why one antidepressant might be highly desirable for one person and not recommended for another.

Occasionally tricyclics may complicate specific heart problems. It is for this reason that your doctor should be aware of any heart condition that you may have. Other side effects may include blurred vision, dry mouth, constipation, weight gain, dizziness, increased sweating, difficulty urinating, changes in sexual desire, decrease in sexual ability, muscle twitches, fatigue, and weakness. Not all tricyclic medications produce all side effects, and not everybody gets them. Some side effects will disappear quickly, while others may remain for the length of treatment.

Some side effects are similar to symptoms of depression such as fatigue and constipation. For this reason, you or your family should discuss all symptoms that you are experiencing with your doctor. These discussions may lead to a change in the medication or dosage.

Tricyclics also may interact with thyroid hormone, antihypertensive medications, oral contraceptives, some blood coagulants, some sleeping medications, antipsychotic medications, diuretics, antihistamines, aspirin, bicarbonate of soda, vitamin C, alcohol, and tobacco.

Especially concerning is that an overdose of antidepressants is serious and potentially lethal and requires immediate medical attention. Symptoms of an overdose of tricyclic antidepressant medication develop within an hour and may start with rapid heartbeat, dilated pupils, flushed face, and agitation, and progress to confusion, loss of consciousness, seizures, irregular heart beats, cardiorespiratory collapse, and death.

Side effects of SSRI's

The most common side effects of SSRI's are sexual dysfunction. Other side effects are gastrointestinal problems such as constipation or diarrhea, headache, insomnia, anxiety, and agitation. Because of potentially serious interaction between these medications and monoamine oxidase inhibitors, it is advisable to stop taking one medication from 2 - 4 weeks before starting the other, depending on the specific medications involved. In addition, some SSRIs have been found to affect metabolism of certain other medications in the liver, creating possible drug interactions.

Side effects of Monoamine Oxidase Inhibitors

Some side effects of Monoamine Oxidase Inhibitors are similar to those of the other antidepressants. Dizziness and rapid heartbeat are common. These antidepressant medications also react with certain foods such as aged cheese or foods containing monosodium glutamate, known as MSG; and alcoholic beverages like red wines as well as other medications such as over-the-counter cold and allergy preparations, local anesthetics, amphetamines, insulin, some narcotics, and anti-parkinson medications.

Reactions often do not appear for several hours and signs may include severe high blood pressure, headache, nausea, vomiting, rapid heartbeat, possible confusion, psychotic symptoms, seizures, stroke, and coma. Because of the severity of the side effects with certain foods, drinks and medications, patients taking these particular antidepressant medications must closely monitor what is ingested and make every attempt to stay away from restricted foods, drinks, and medications.

The patient should be sure their doctor or pharmacist furnishes a complete list of all foods, beverages, and other medications that should be avoided.

General precautions when taking Antidepressants

It is important to tell your doctors and dentist about all medications that you are currently using. Your list should include prescription medications, over-the-counter medications and preparations as well as alcohol.

Antidepressants should be taken only in the amount prescribed and should be kept in a secure place away from children. When used with proper care, following doctors' instructions, antidepressants are extremely useful medications that can reverse the symptoms and misery of a depression and help you feel like yourself again.

Chapter 9

Treatment

The treatment options vary depending on the symptoms and severity the patient is experiencing and treatment for Crohn's is limited to a wide array of drugs or surgery. Patients with minimal disease activity, mild or no symptoms and whose disease is in remission may not need treatment. Patients with moderate symptoms may require only drug treatment while severe symptoms may require surgery to correct.

There is no medication that can cure Crohn's disease. Patients will typically experience periods of relapse followed by periods of remission lasting months to years. During relapses, symptoms of abdominal pain, diarrhea, and rectal bleeding worsen. During remissions, these symptoms improve or can go away all together. Remissions usually occur because of treatment with medications or surgery, but occasionally they occur spontaneously, that is, without any treatment.

Since there is no cure for the disease, the goals of treatment are to induce remissions, maintain remissions, minimize side effects of treatment and improve the quality of life.

Treatment of Crohn's disease and ulcerative colitis with medications is similar though not always identical.

Drug Treatment

There are many drugs with many side effects to treat Crohn's disease. We will discuss those drugs in the next section. Currently there are several different drugs in various stages of development for the treatment of Crohn's disease.

Nicotine Treatment

In marked contrast to ulcerative colitis patients, a higher proportion of Crohn's patients smoke and it appears that continued smoking is a forecaster of post surgical recurrence of Crohn's. This data suggests that smoking may be a co-factor predisposing the development of Crohn's and having a preventive effect in ulcerative colitis. These tendencies and data are not fully understood.

Due to the overall health risks of smoking, doctors have been reluctant to fully accept this data as being reliable. Recently more attention has been devoted to understanding the relationship between smoking Crohn's disease. Many ulcerative colitis patients have reported that their symptoms began after quitting smoking. From that, one question that has inspired considerable work has been whether nicotine is responsible for the apparently protective effect of in ulcerative colitis.

Two articles were published in The New England Journal of Medicine studying the potential therapeutic benefit of nicotine patches, normally used to help people stop smoking, to induce remission of active ulcerative colitis and to maintain its remission. The patches were helpful in some patients in the induction of remission but were not helpful in the maintenance of remission. Most non smoking patients in the studies suffered some side effects from the nicotine, including nausea, vomiting, lightheadedness, headache and sleeplessness. More work needs to be done to clarify the role of nicotine in therapy of ulcerative colitis.

Tumor Necrosis Factor

When the immune system is activated resulting in inflammation, many chemical messengers are released. These chemical messengers are produced by the cells of the immune system and are called cytokines. These cytokines interact with other cells encouraging them to become activated and thus make the inflammation worse. Tumor Necrosis Factor is one of the most important cytokines involved in this process. The term Tumor Necrosis Factor refers to one of its actions, which led to its discovery

At the onset of an infection, Tumor Necrosis Factor frequently plays an important role in helping the immune system respond promptly and effectively. It is believed, however; that excessive and inappropriate production of Tumor Necrosis Factor may be an important contributory factor in the development of several diseases characterized by inflammation and activation of the immune system such as multiple sclerosis, rheumatoid arthritis and others. Therapies that are being developed for these diseases may also be useful for treating Crohn's disease. There has been considerable publicity recently given to the new data about the treatment of Crohn's disease with antibodies against Tumor Necrosis Factor.

Various strategies have been used to evaluate the importance of Tumor Necrosis Factor in Crohn's disease and ulcerative colitis. Though some data does support a role it has been difficult to convincingly demonstrate that there is excessive production of Tumor Necrosis Factor in either disease. The available data seems to suggest that Tumor Necrosis Factor may be of more importance in Crohn's disease than ulcerative colitis. The fact that the new anti-Tumor Necrosis Factor treatments seem effective in some patients is the best evidence that Tumor Necrosis Factor is important in the disease process of Crohn's disease.

The treatment itself consists of an antibody, which is a protein that neutralizes the action of Tumor Necrosis Factor. Originally, a mouse produced the antibody when it was injected with human Tumor Necrosis Factor. The immune system of the mouse recognized the foreign nature of the human Tumor Necrosis Factor and produced antibodies against it. One of these mouse produced antibodies was humanized so that it would be less likely to provoke an adverse reaction when injected into a human. From these experiments, there have been two antibodies that have been used to treat Crohn's disease.

The biotechnology company Centecor developed the first antibody, named cA2. The cA2 antibody was initially used in the treatment of severe infection but more recently it has been evaluated for the treatment of rheumatoid arthritis. Because of promising results in the arthritis studies a group of Dutch physicians gave the antibody to a child with severe Crohn's disease there was a dramatic response to the drug. This encouraged more comprehensive studies of the effectiveness of the cA2 antibody to treat Crohn's disease in Europe and the United States, which are currently on-going.

The second anti-Tumor Necrosis Factor antibody has been developed by the biotechnology company British Biotechnology and is called CDP571.

The anti-Tumor Necrosis Factor treatment works by having the antibodies block the actions of Tumor Necrosis Factor. The fact that it is so effective in some patients has raised the question whether it is having some additional effects on the immune system. This remains concern remains to be clarified. The antibody is given by intravenous infusion and cannot be given by mouth and it is not clear whether it can be given safely to the same patient more than once. If the medication can be given repeatedly to a patient, it remains to be seen whether it will continue to have a beneficial effect or whether resistance to the antibodies will emerge.

Like most treatments and medications for Crohn's disease patients, anti-Tumor Necrosis Factor medication does not seem to work in all patients. Recent studies show that most patients who received the treatment had a beneficial response about half actually went into remission. However, in those patients who have a response to the medication, the effect is temporary, lasting at best several months.

The treatment will only be available as part of formal clinical studies for the next few years. If it continues to have positive results and becomes available as a standard therapy in the next few years it is likely to be expensive. The most important aspect of the tests and its use though is that it implies that Tumor Necrosis Factor does indeed seem to have an important role in the development of inflammation of Crohn's disease in a significant percentage of patients.

Crohn's disease patients with active disease despite therapy with steroids seem to be the most likely candidates for the tests. Having the disease and active symptoms are a prerequisite for enrollment in the studies. Those patients who may particularly be suitable for the anti-Tumor Necrosis Factor therapy are those who cannot tolerate 6-mercaptopurine (6-MP) or in whom 6-mercaptopurine has not worked or have just been started on 6-mercaptopurine and a therapeutic effect is not expected for several months. Currently, the anti-Tumor Necrosis Factor antibodies are only available as part of formal studies at present.

Alternative treatments available at present

The best-tested and most effective medications at present are 6-MP and methotrexate. Other medications are also being developed which block the action of Tumor Necrosis Factor, which may be useful in the treatment of Crohn's disease in the future.

Interleukin-10 (IL-10) therapy for Crohn's disease

IL-10 is another cytokine like Tumor Necrosis Factor. Like other Tumor Necrosis Factor medications, IL-10 suppresses the immune system and is presently also being studied in the treatment of Crohn's disease. The medical community and patients eagerly await the results of this study.

There is some evidence that fish oil containing eicosapentaenoic acid has anti- inflammatory properties that may be useful in the treatment of Crohn's disease and rheumatoid arthritis. Fish oil may also be helpful in preventing cardiovascular disease. On the downside, patient acceptance of fish oil therapy has been poor because of the indigestion and bad breath associated with the therapy. A recent Italian study used coated capsules containing fish oil and showed evidence of benefit in preventing recurrences of Crohn's disease with minimal side-effects. These capsules are not widely available at present.

In the interim various fish oil preparations containing eicosapentaenoic acid are available from pharmacies and health food stores which may be of therapeutic benefit despite the possible side-effect of increased susceptibility to bleeding. If you don't want to take fish oil because of the side effects, simply eat more fish.

Many patients require treatment with more than one medication to adequately control their symptoms. Frequently, several different combinations are tried before the best one is found. Once symptoms are brought under control then attempts are made to reduce the medications to a minimum.

At this point in time because there is no cure for Crohn's disease it is strongly advised for patients to continue taking their medications to keep them in remission. The reason for this, which is supported by some studies, is that it is much easier to keep a patient in remission rather than treat a flare of the disease.

Surgery for Crohn's disease patients

Unlike ulcerative colitis, there is no surgical cure for Crohn's disease. Physicians use the phrases "minimal surgery" and "surgery avoidance" when discussing surgical options for Crohn's disease treatment. Because new Crohn's disease lesions can appear after previously diseased areas have been removed, many surgeons feel that surgery in Crohn's patients just leads to more surgery. Also, some of the diseased tissue may be functionally useful.

Surgery for Crohn's disease patients usually is resection of the small intestines or colon whereby severely affected portions of the organ are removed and the healthy ends are sewn together. This in no way prevents inflammation from recurring later and is generally performed only when the inflammation is unable to be controlled by medical therapy.

There is some evidence that some 5-ASA drugs, especially Pentasa, may be useful in preventing disease recurrence after surgery. Some experts use 6-MP following surgery in patients with a high risk of recurrence and there is a trial in progress to see if it works in this setting. There is also some limited evidence that metronidazole may be helpful in preventing disease recurrence following surgery.

Smoking is associated with recurrent disease following surgery in Crohn's disease patients. Clearly, and without question, Crohn's disease patients must be strongly encouraged to stop smoking.

Surgery is the last ditch effort to treat patients with Crohn's disease.

Surgery for ulcerative colitis patients

Since drug treatments are ineffective in about 20 percent of ulcerative colitis patients, these patients must have their colons removed due to debilitating symptoms. The colon may also be removed because of the threat of cancer. Removal of the colon permanently cures the ulcerative colitis and usually all related symptoms.

Colectomy with ileorectal anastomosis

This procedure is one that is performed to cure ulcerative colitis or colon cancer. It is not a cure Crohn's disease. This procedure involves removing the whole of the colon and joining the ilium to the top of the rectum, known as anastomosed. That is why it is called a colectomy with an ileorectal anastomosis.

It may be necessary for the patient to stay in hospital for 6 - 8 days with most people getting back to a normal life in about six weeks. Strenuous exercise, such as lifting heavy weights, should be avoided for about 3 months. Following this procedure, most patients will go to the toilet 3 or 4 times a day and the stools may be softer than before. If a person finds that they need to go

143

more often, Imodium tablets can be taken. Imodium slows down and relaxes the bowel. Imodium is not addictive.

After recovery from this procedure, some find that certain types of food upset their bowel and are best avoided while others eat whatever they want when they want to with no adverse side effects. People differ greatly but beer, spicy foods, raw vegetables and fruit are often mentioned as causing loose bowel motions. Each person has to find out what suits them and food will be discussed later in this handbook.

Patients who have had a colectomy with ileorectal nastomosis will still have their rectum. Polyps, which are small swellings, arising from the lining of the bowel, may continue to develop in the rectum. It is therefore important that the rectum be examined regularly. This is usually done as an outpatient procedure every six months.

Proctocolectomy

A permanent proctocolectomy with ileostomy is rarely done for polyposis, but is the ultimate cure for ulcerative colitis or colon cancer. This procedure involves removing the entire colon, rectum and anus. The ileum is then brought out onto the abdomen where it protrudes about an inch. This is called an ileostomy. It is stitched into place so there is no need to worry about it falling back inside.

The body's feces will come out of the ileostomy into a bag that is securely stuck onto the skin of the abdomen and which is worn under the clothes. This bag is discrete and usually not seen or noticeable.

With an ileostomy it is not possible to control when it will act but it is possible to control the emptying or changing of the bag. The stoma care nurse will provide support and education about the care of the ileostomy.

It is usually necessary to stay in hospital for about 2 weeks. The patient's return to normal activity begins about 6 - 8 weeks after the procedure and the majority of individuals with an ileostomy will lead a normal life. Strenuous activity should be avoided for about 3 months; however, activities such as swimming do not need to be avoided. Some people find it best to avoid certain foods, especially those that are fibrous and pithy, for example, oranges, because they can lead to obstruction of the small bowel.

Patients with an ileostomy are usually seen by their doctor on a yearly basis.

A restorative proctocolectomy is a procedure that involves removing the colon and the rectum, but not the anus. An artificial rectum, called a J-pouch, is made out of the lower end of the ileum. The J-pouch is jointed to the anus so bowel actions can be controlled in the normal way. The J-pouch stores the feces until the person goes to the lavatory in the usual way. This operation is usually performed in two steps.

In the first step, the colon and rectum are removed and the J-pouch is made and joined to the anus. This procedure is quite complicated so it is sometimes necessary to allow the new J-pouch time to rest while it heals. This is done by creating a temporary ileostomy above the J-pouch, which means that stools have to be collected in a bag, which is worn outside the body, on the abdomen.

The average stay in hospital for this procedure is about 10 - 12 days. The patients return to light work is usually possible between four to six weeks. Strenuous activity should be avoided for about 3 months; however, activities such as swimming do not need to be avoided.

145

After approximately 2 months your doctor will perform the second step of this procedure. When the J-pouch has healed, the ileostomy is closed by a second surgical procedure so that stools are again passed from the anus in the usual way. The average stay in hospital for this step is approximately 4 - 6 days.

Sometimes it is possible to do the operation without creating a temporary ileostomy. This option should be discussed with the surgeon.

In the early stages after the procedure, most people pass soft stool. When the body finally adjusts to the ileostomy, most people find they need to go to the lavatory between 4 and 6 times a day. The stool will be the consistency of porridge and it should be no problem to hold on for a while after feeling the urge to go. In some cases, the patient may need to go at night and few may feel more confident if they wear a small pad in case of any minor leakage.

Some patients find that certain types of food upset their bowels but they find out which by trial and error. Foods that are fibrous or pithy, for example, oranges, should be eaten with care or avoided as they may lead to the bowel becoming obstructed.

If the bowel actions are too frequent or diarrhea is experienced, an adjustment to the diet or the need to take Imodium may become necessary. Imodium slows down and relaxes the bowel and is not addictive.

The patient will usually be examined by their once a year.

Emotional state and coping with surgery

There is a certain amount of stress involved with going through a surgical procedure. To that end, the object for a Crohnie is to have as few surgical procedures as possible. For obvious reasons then, surgery is recommended only for a minority of patients with Crohn's disease and then only in a last ditch effort to correct the problems when the disease can not be controlled by medications. When surgery is needed, it poses some immediate risk to the patient, but in the appropriate circumstances this risk should be outweighed by the expected benefit.

With modern surgery and pre and postoperative care, the dangers of serious complications from surgery are quite low. This does not, however, eliminate the stress involved with the surgical procedure and some additional problems of adjustment that the patient must now deal with along with coping with a disease that they probably don't fully understand. These newfound problems can be more easily dealt with, thereby reducing overall stress of the situation, by being informed.

As with any surgical procedure, there can be complications. The most common complication of the operations mentioned above is inflammation of the J-pouch, called pouchitis. Symptoms include pain, bloating, and diarrhea. Most patients can control this by irrigating the J-pouch with saline solution and taking antibiotics. In a few cases, a diagnosis of Crohn's disease is confirmed in patients thought originally to be suffering from ulcerative colitis.

Problems with the nipple valve in a continent ileostomy can cause leakage of stool and an inability to insert the catheter. About 10% of patients require a second operation to repair the nipple valve.

Acupuncture & Crohn's Disease

In 1979 the World Health Organization listed 40 major diseases in which the patients could experience relief by acupuncture. Diseases of the digestive system were included on that list.

Acupuncture has been successfully used in China to treat a multitude of different illnesses that can be traced back at least 2,500 years. The general theory of acupuncture is based on the premise that there are patterns of energy flow through the body, known as Qi, which are essential for good health. Disruptions of this flow are believed to be responsible for disease and it has been theorized that acupuncture may correct imbalances of flow at identifiable points close to the skin.

Acupuncture has also been shown to cause the brain to release endorphins and encephalons, which are the body's natural painkillers, as well as boosting the immune system and providing a calming of the nervous system.

The practice of acupuncture to treat identifiable disease conditions in American medicine was rare before the visit of President Richard M. Nixon to China in 1972. Since that time, there has been an explosion of interest in the United States and Europe in the application of the technique of acupuncture.

What is acupuncture?

Acupuncture is a series of procedures involving stimulation of anatomical locations on or in the skin by a variety of techniques. There are a variety of approaches to diagnosis and treatment in American acupuncture those incorporate medical traditions from China, Japan, Korea, and other countries.

The most thoroughly studied mechanism of stimulation of acupuncture points employs penetration of the skin by thin, solid, metallic needles, which are manipulated manually or by electrical stimulation.

Side Effects of Acupuncture

The most common serious injury reported from the needles of acupuncture has been accidental puncture of the lung. This injury results in a partial collapse of the lung called pneumothorax. The most common infection reported from acupuncture treatments is viral hepatitis. Other side effects include bacterial infections locally at the site of needle insertion in the skin and elsewhere in the body.

Generally, side effects seem to relate to poor hygiene and training of the acupuncturist.

Information for this section was furnished, in part, by The National Institutes of Health of the United States Government.

Hypnotherapy/Psychotherapy

All physical diseases including diabetes, cancer, heart disease, Crohn's disease and ulcerative colitis have been helped with hypnotherapy and psychotherapy. The power of suggestion and mental imagery is a tool all too often overlooked in the treatment of Crohn's disease.

Since Crohn's disease is a stress related disease, hypnotherapy and psychotherapy are both excellent aids to help control emotional stress.

A controlled study in Europe involving 266 patients suffering from Crohn's disease revealed that psychotherapy is an important element in the treatment of this disease. The researchers found that psychotherapy can improve the therapeutic possibilities of drugs, diet and surgery. Psychotherapy combined with relaxation and removal of stress were considered along with the personality of the patient before the outbreak of the disease. It was suggested that unknown emotional

149

conflicts such as depression, mental lability and anorexia may influence the course of the disease.

Psychotherapy of Crohn's disease Zur Psychotherapie des M. Crohn. Feiereis H Langenbecks Arch Chir 1984, 364 p407-11

Chapter 10

Medications

Because no medical cure for Crohn's disease exists, the goals of medical treatment are to suppress the inflammatory areas, permit healing of the tissue and relieve certain symptoms that are experienced during an attack. Most patients with Crohn's disease will experience periodic increases in activity of the disease when symptoms of abdominal pain, fever, diarrhea, and rectal bleeding worsen. Medications are then used to bring the active disease into remission. Medications for the treatment of active Crohn's disease include aminosalicylate preparations, corticosteroids, antibiotics, and medications that suppress body immunity. The decision regarding which treatments are used is based on the location and the severity of the disease. Patients with advanced disease causing persistent bowel obstruction, abscess, and fistulae may need surgery.

The groups of drugs mentioned above that form the mainstay of treatment for Crohn's disease today are:

- **Aminosalicylates**: aspirin-like drugs, which include sulfasalazine and mesalamine, given both orally and rectally (5-ASA).
- **Corticosteroids**: prednisone and methylprednisolone, available orally and rectally.

- **Immune modifiers**: azathioprine, 6MP, methotrexate.
- **Antibiotics**: metronidazole, ampicillin, ciprofloxacin, and others.

(A complete list of the above medications and their side effects is contained in the index at the end of this book)

Aminosalicylates

5-aminosalicylic acid (5-ASA), also called mesalamine, is an anti-inflammatory drug used in treating Crohn's disease. 5-ASA has a similar chemical structure to aspirin, but has a 5-amino group in place of aspirin's acetyl group (aspirin is acetylsalicylic acid).

Pure unmodified 5-ASA is easily absorbed in the upper gastrointestinal tract. To enable its delivery to the lower gastrointestinal tract where it is needed it must be chemically modified or packaged. Different 5-ASA drugs are formulated to allow delivery to different locations. Because of the chemical similarities to aspirin, patients allergic to aspirin should not take 5-ASA drugs.

The sulfa-free 5-ASA (mesalamine) compounds have fewer side effects than Azulfidine, and also do not impair male fertility. They are mostly safe medications for long term use and are well tolerated.

Patients allergic to aspirin should avoid 5-ASA (mesalamine) compounds because they are chemically similar to aspirin.

Rare kidney inflammation has been reported with the use of 5-ASA compounds. These compounds should be used with caution in patients with known kidney disease. It also is recommended that blood tests of kidney function be measured before starting and periodically during treatment.

Rare instances of acute worsening of diarrhea, cramps, and abdominal pain which is at times accompanied by fever, rash, and malaise may occur. This reaction is believed to represent an allergy to the 5-ASA compound.

Corticosteroids

Corticostoeroids and other anti inflammatory agents are used to control symptoms and to attempt to induce remission. When 5-ASA drugs fail or when symptoms are more severe, the next therapeutic step usually involves steroids, which are very powerful anti-inflammatory drugs.

These medications are available in oral, enema, or suppository forms. The topical forms are useful in treating distal colitis the oral forms are useful for achieving remission in mild to moderate active Crohn's disease and ulcerative colitis. They are NOT useful for continued use in order to maintain a remission. The oral forms can, however, be effective in suppressing active Crohn's disease to the point where it appears to be in remission.

Steroids are a group of hormones with similar chemical structures. They are normally produced by your adrenal glands, located on top of your kidneys, and your reproductive organs (ovaries and testicles). Steroids help control metabolism, inflammation, immune function, salt and water balance, development of sexual characteristics and your ability to withstand the stress of illness and injury.

Because of the serious potential side effects and problems that can be caused by taking steroids, it is very important that your Doctor closely supervise any steroid therapy. People taking Corticosteroids have developed Kaposi's sarcoma, a form of cancer.

Common side effects include rounding of the face, known as moon face. Increase in the size of fat pads on the upper back and back of the neck, known as a buffalo hump. Acne. Increased appetite with weight gain. Increased body hair. Osteoporosis, especially in women. Compression fractures in vertebrae. Diabetes. Hypertension. Cataracts and glaucoma. Increased susceptibility to infections. Weakness of arm, leg, shoulder, and pelvic muscles. Personality changes including depression, irritability, nervousness, and insomnia. Suicidal tendencies are not uncommon for patients who take steroids.

Children's growth may be affected, even by small doses of steroids.

As mentioned, steroid drugs can cause osteoporosis. For many years it was thought that only high (20mg / day or higher) doses of steroids were a problem, more recent studies have shown that chronic use of low oral doses as little as 7.5 mg / day can cause significant though gradual bone loss.

Steroids reduce the amount of calcium the body absorbs from food and increase calcium loss through the kidneys. These actions result in a tendency for the level of calcium in the blood to fall. To prevent this condition the body responds by producing increased amounts of the parathyroid hormone. Parathyroid hormone is released to remove calcium from storage in the bone and restore a normal level. In addition steroids also cause bone breakdown directly.

The best strategy is to avoid potential bone loss entirely is by using the lowest effective dose of the steroid. Also use topical steroids if possible instead of systemic steroids by mouth.

It is highly recommended that either before or at the very start of steroid therapy, the patient should ideally be given a bone density test, especially of the lower spine and the thighbone near where it meets the pelvis. This test should be repeated every 6 - 12 months to monitor the effectiveness of preventive measures and, if necessary, to modify the course of treatment.

These tests are important because a serious complication of steroid therapy is avascular necrosis of the hip. This results in death of the bone in the hip joint resulting in arthritis and severe pain. Fortunately, it is a rare complication.

Patients on steroids should perform regular weight-bearing exercise, preferably for 30 - 60 minutes a day as this can help prevent bone loss. Patients should not smoke or drink more than moderate amounts of alcohol as these are associated with increased rates of bone loss.

To help slow or eliminate the possibility of bone loss, everyone who must take corticosteroids should consume at least 1,500 mg of calcium and 800 IU (International Units) of vitamin D a day, either through diet or supplements. Vitamin D is needed to enhance the body's ability to absorb calcium and use it to build bone.

Consideration should be given to hormone replacement therapy in woman who is post menopause. Women who have not yet reached menopause whose periods become irregular or stop while on steroids should take oral contraceptives unless there is a medical reason for not taking them. For men on steroids consideration should be given to measuring their testosterone level and, if found to be low, given testosterone replacement.

Corticosteroids suppress the activity of the adrenal glands, which must be restored gradually when the drug is discontinued. This requires gradual tapering of the steroid. Most physicians will not taper long-term steroid

155

users faster than roughly 1 mg per week or 5 mg per month. For short-term users, dosage may be lowered at a faster rate, such as 5 - 10 mg per week.

Withdrawal symptoms can occur when the dosage is lowered too quickly. These may include fever, malaise, and joint pains. Since these can also be symptoms of IBD, it is often difficult to tell whether they are the result of insufficient steroid levels, or a true relapse of the disease.

If symptoms begin to return during tapering, standard procedure is to return to a slightly higher dose, which is maintained until symptoms subside. Tapering may then be resumed at a slower rate.

If you've been taking steroids for any length of time, it would be in your best interest to invest in and wear a MEDIC-ALERT necklace or bracelet. On it, indicate the quantity and duration of steroid use. If you require emergency surgery, this information can be of vital importance since you'll need to be administered additional steroids. Your body isn't capable of producing enough steroids on its own to help survive the stress.

Increasing the period of time between steroid doses can allow the adrenal glands to recover somewhat. Alternate day therapy could be how this is done. Alternate day therapy is simply taking double the daily dose every other day. Due to the duration and severity of the effects of taking steroids this can have the same therapeutic results with fewer side effects.

Immune Modifiers

Immunosuppressives, also referred to as immune modifiers, such as 6-mercaptopurine (6-MP or purinethol) or azathioprine (imuran) are increasingly used in treating more severe Crohn's disease that does not respond to 5-ASA therapy and short term steroid therapy.

The most frequent use of these drugs is in the context of inability to reduce the steroid dosages in steroid dependent patients without causing a disease flare. Physicians without significant experience in their use can be reluctant to try them because they can have extreme side effects. Generally these side effects occur at higher doses than are used in the treatment of Crohn's disease. However, the emphatic opinion of most physician experts in the management of Crohn's disease is that they are significantly safer and more effective than long term use of high dose steroids.

The side effects that occur in a small minority of the patients who take them can include various blood problems, bone marrow suppression, extensive immune suppression, kidney damage, liver damage and others. There is no convincing evidence that they lead to the development of cancer at the doses used in treating Crohn's patients.

Antibiotics

It is very important to use antibiotics appropriately. Antibiotics are powerful drugs used to treat certain illnesses. Antibiotics do not cure everything, and unnecessary antibiotics can even be harmful. Basically, there are two main types of germs that cause most infections. These are viruses and bacteria.

Each time you take an antibiotic, bacteria are killed. Sometimes bacteria may be resistant or become resistant. Resistant bacteria do not respond to the antibiotics and continue to cause infection.

Each time you take an antibiotic unnecessarily or improperly, you increase your chance of developing drug-resistant bacteria. So it is really important to take antibiotics only when necessary. Because of these resistant bacteria, some diseases that used to be easy to treat are now becoming nearly impossible to treat.

The following facts are what you should know about antibiotics.

Antibiotics don't work against colds and flu, and those unnecessary antibiotics can be harmful.

Talk to your Doctor about antibiotics and find out about the differences between viruses and bacteria. Ask and understand when antibiotics should and shouldn't be used.

If you do get an antibiotic, be sure to take it exactly as prescribed. This will help decrease the development of resistant bacteria.

Antibiotic resistance is particularly dangerous for children, but it can occur in adults as well.

One final note is that taking antibiotics appropriately will help prevent having to take more dangerous and more costly medications. If you use antibiotics appropriately you can avoid developing drug resistance. Just take your medicine exactly as your Doctor prescribes it.

Medications with special side effects

Below are some medications that have some special side effects or will have effects on the body and you should pay special attention to them. Some of these medications are listed in the Medication Index, but because of the serious or special attributes of the medication, they have been included in this section as well.

Sulfasalazine

Sulfasalazine (Azulfidine, Azulfidine EN-Tabs in the US; Salazopyrin EN-Tabs, SAS in Canada; Salazosulfapyridine, Salicylazosulfapyridine), is the "staple" drug generally first prescribed for Crohn's patients. It is taken by mouth and is intended to first reduce inflammation of the intestinal lining and then to maintain remission in mild to moderate cases. Sulfasalazine is a combination of Sulfapyridine and a compound of 5-aminosalicylic acid. Intestinal bacteria, making the 5-ASA available in the terminal ileum and colon break the bond between the two. A significant amount of the Sulfapyridine component is absorbed, metabolized by the liver, and excreted in urine. Side effects are experienced by some patients and can include nausea, heartburn, headache, dizziness, anemia, and skin rashes. It is also known to cause a reduced sperm count in men, but only for the duration of treatment. It may also turn urine a bright orange-yellow color. The side effects generally result from the Sulfapyridine component. Because of this, there are efforts to develop formulations of 5-ASA, which do not contain Sulfapyridine or other sulfa drugs.

Azulfidine

Azulfidine was developed in the 1930's for the treatment of rheumatoid arthritis. During clinical trials in the 1940's, arthritis patients who also suffered from irritable bowel disease reported improvements in their conditions and symptoms while taking the medication. This led to its current use as the mainstay irritable bowel disease treatment.

For active disease initially, 1 gram every 6 - 8 hours is taken by mouth. Reducing the dosage to 500 mg every 6 - 12 hours may lessen adverse effects. Maintenance dose is usually 500 mg every 6 hours, adjusted to patient response and tolerance. Total doses of more than 4 g/day may increase the risk of adverse effects and toxicity but some patients may benefit from taking up to 6 g/day. Azulfadine is generally taken with a full glass of water after meals or with food to minimize indigestion. However, when indigestion is a problem, enteric-coated tablets may be used which are tolerated better.

Asacol (Mesalamine, USA; Mesalazine, Europe)

Asacol is a tablet consisting of 5-ASA Mesalamine compound surrounded by an acrylic resin coating which dissolves at pH greater than 7. Asacol is essentially "Azulfidine without the sulfa". The resin coating protects the 5-ASA from being absorbed as it passes through the stomach and the small intestine. When the tablet reaches the terminal ileum and the colon, where the pH is typically greater than 7, the resin coating dissolves, thus releasing the active 5-ASA drug into the colon.

Asacol is effective in inducing remission in patients with mild to moderate ulcerative colitis. It also is effective when used long term to maintain remissions. Some studies have shown that Asacol also is effective in treating active Crohn's disease, as well as in maintaining remission.

The recommended dose of Asacol to induce remission is two 400-mg tablets three times daily (total of 2.4 g/day). Two tablets of Asacol twice daily (1.6 g/day) is recommended for maintaining remission. Occasionally, the maintenance dose is higher.

160

As with Azulfidine, the benefits of Asacol are dose related. If patients do not respond to 2.4 g/day of Asacol, the dose is frequently increased to 3.6 g/day (sometimes even higher) to induce remission. If patients fail to respond to the higher doses of Asacol, then other alternatives such as Corticosteroids are considered.

Salofalk (Mesalazine, Europe)

Similar to Asacol but dissolves at pH greater than 6.

Balsalazide

Another 5-ASA drug that uses a variant on Sulfasalazine's delivery mechanism. Balsalazide contains 5-ASA joined to an inert vehicle. This combination passes through the stomach and upper ileum. Intestinal bacteria then break it down in the terminal ileum, making 5-ASA available in the terminal ileum and colon.

Rowasa

Rowasa is 5-ASA in enema form and is effective in treating distal ulcerative colitis, which is simply the disease affecting the lower part of the colon, near the rectum, and the rectum itself. One enema contains 4 grams of 5-ASA.

Rowasa also comes in suppository form for treating proctitis. Each suppository contains 500 mg of 5-ASA.

Pentasa

Pentasa is a capsule consisting of the 5-ASA compound inside small time-release spheres. It also is sulfa free. As the capsule travels down the intestines, the 5-ASA inside the spheres is slowly released into the intestines. Unlike Asacol, the active drug 5-ASA in Pentasa is released into the small intestine as well as the colon. Therefore, Pentasa can be effective in treating inflammation in the small intestine, and is currently the most commonly used 5-ASA compound for treating mild to moderate Crohn's disease in the small intestine.

Patients with Crohn's disease occasionally undergo surgery to relieve small intestinal obstruction, drain infected abscesses, or remove fistulae. Usually, the diseased portions of the intestines are removed during surgery. After successful surgery, patients can be free of disease and symptoms for some time. In many patients, however, Crohn's disease eventually will return. Pentasa helps maintain remission and reduces the chances of the recurrence of Crohn's disease after surgery.

In the treatment of Crohn's ileitis or ileocolitis, the dose of Pentasa usually is four 250 mg capsules four times daily (total of 16 capsules or 4 g/day). For maintenance of remission in patients after surgery, the dose of Pentasa is between 2 to 4 grams of Pentasa daily.

Olsalazine Sodium (Dipentum)

Olsalazine is a drug that uses a different mechanism to deliver 5-ASA to the terminal ileum and colon. Whereas Sulfasalazine links a 5-ASA molecule with a Sulfapyridine molecule, Olsalazine links two 5-ASA molecules. This compound passes through the stomach and upper ileum. Intestinal bacteria then break it down in the terminal ileum, making 5-ASA available there and also in the colon.

The major side effect is watery diarrhea, seen in many patients. Patients with Crohns' affecting the entire colon seem especially susceptible. Increased cramping and audible bowel sounds are also commonly reported.

162

The usual dose of Dipentum is 500 mg by mouth twice a day.

Prednisone

One of the steroids produced by the outer portion of the adrenal glands is called cortisone. It normally helps regulate the body's salt and water balance and reduces inflammation. Introduced in 1955, Prednisone is the man-made replica of cortisone. The adrenal glands normally produce an amount of steroids equivalent to about 5 mg of Prednisone a day. When prescribed in doses that exceed natural levels, Prednisone suppresses inflammation and can help treat a variety of diseases such as severe allergies or skin problems, asthma, arthritis, ulcerative colitis, and Crohn's disease. Prednisone is also used to help prevent rejection of organ transplants.

Prednisone is the generic form; some common brand names are Deltasone, Meticorten, Orasone, and SK-Prednisone.

Prednisone is not the same as the dangerous anabolic steroids used by weight lifters to increase muscle mass. It is not a sex hormone like testosterone or estrogen and does not cause sexual dysfunction. Prednisone is not addictive. It does not cause drowsiness and in the usual doses will not affect driving or working. There is no special food interaction and mild alcohol consumption is not a problem while taking Prednisone.

Prednisolone

Prednisolone is classified as a synthetic adrenal corticosteroid.

Hydrocortisone

Hydrocortisone is another name for the steroid hormone Cortisol, more especially used to refer to preparations of this hormone used medicinally. Hydrocortisone, introduced in 1952, is more potent than cortisone with respect to medicinal metabolic and anti-inflammatory effects. Like cortisone, it is used to treat inflammatory and rheumatoid diseases, and allergies. Low-potency hydrocortisone, available over the counter, is used to treat skin irritations.

Entocort

Entocort is a corticosteroid mainly used in the treatment of Crohn's disease. Corticosteroids have potent anti-inflammatory properties and are used in a wide variety of inflammatory conditions. Entocort decreases the inflammation in the small intestine and the first part of the large intestine.

Budesonide

Budesonide is currently in beta testing. It is a steroid that is processed by the liver so that there are less severe side effects. Oral and enema forms are available, depending upon the location of the disease to be treated. Its role compared to the more established steroid agents has yet to be defined. The impression of many is that though it may be safer it may also be less effective.

Adreno-cortico-tropic hormone

Adreno-cortico-tropic hormone is a drug that stimulates the adrenal gland to release cortisone. It is seldom used any more.

Methotrexate (Folex, Mexate in the US)

Like the other immunosuppressants, Methotrexate may have some benefit in treating active Crohn's disease. Methotrexate has not been used as extensively as Azathioprine or 6-MP but there is increasing data that it may be useful. Methotrexate may be a useful option in patients who are intolerant of Azathioprine or 6-MP. Because of the occurrence of liver disease in patients taking Methotrexate over a sustained period careful monitoring of liver function is necessary. Patients should not drink alcohol while taking Methotrexate.

Methotrexate should not be used in pregnancy and patients taking Methotrexate should not get pregnant.

Cyclosporine

Cyclosporine is another immunosuppressant drug that was originally and is still used extensively for preventing rejection of organ transplants such as kidney and liver transplants.

Though initial hopes were high that it would be a very good drug for severe and complicated Crohn's the results have been somewhat disappointing.

In severe Crohn's, particularly complicated by fistulas, there is data that high dose intravenous Cyclosporine may be useful in the short term. Low dose therapy for maintenance of remission does not seem to be effective and has unacceptable side effects.

In severe ulcerative colitis, particularly when a patient is on the threshold of requiring urgent surgery, there has been some success with Cyclosporine in inducing a remission. These patients are generally treated simultaneously with high dose steroids and are started on 6-MP or Azathioprine. After 3 - 6 months of

165

therapy, when 6-MP or Azathioprine has hopefully become effective, Cyclosporine is stopped and simultaneously steroids are reduced and stopped if possible. This approach seems to be effective in the short term with a significant proportion of patients with severe ulcerative colitis. Unfortunately, a significant proportion of these patients subsequently have surgery because of their inability to maintain remission.

Flagyl (Metronidazole)

Flagyl is an antibiotic effective use most frequently for treating vaginal infections. There is, however; some evidence albeit of it anecdotal rather than from formal studies, that it is useful in treating Crohn's. Some studies have shown that it has an anti-inflammatory action on Crohn's disease that is at least as effective as Sulfasalazine. The mechanism of this action is unknown, and it has not been found in other antibiotics having the same antibiotic spectrum. Flagyl appears to be particularly effective in the treatment of Crohn's in the colon.

The medication has been found to be effective against anaerobic bacteria and certain parasites Anaerobic bacteria are single-cell living organisms that thrive in low oxygen environments and can cause disease in the abdomen (bacterial peritonitis), liver (liver abscess), and pelvis (abscess of the ovaries and the fallopian tubes). Giardia lamblia and ameba are parasites that can cause abdominal pain and chronic diarrhea in infected individuals. Flagyl selectively blocks some of the cell functions in these microorganisms, resulting in their elimination.

Though it has been shown to cause cancer in laboratory rodents exposed to very high doses that are much higher than used in humans, there is NO evidence

166

that it has any similar effect in humans. Some patients are unable to tolerate alcohol while taking Flagyl. It is therefore highly recommended that patients avoid alcohol while taking it.

The major side effect of Flagyl is irritation of nerves that can result in permanent nerve damage if the medication is not promptly stopped. The first sign of this problem is usually a sensation of "pins and needles" in the finger tips and toes. The medication should be stopped immediately if the patient experiences this condition.

The biggest issue of Flagyl is that it contains the disclaimer "Crohn's disease is not an approved indication for Metronidazole".

Ciprofloxacin

Ciprofloxacin ("Cipro") is another antibiotic frequently used in the treatment of Crohn's. Many physicians and patients report positive results from a trial of Cipro, although the formal evidence to justify its use is limited. An infrequent side effect of prolonged use is the development of inflammation of tendons, known as tendonitis, which may result in rupture especially of the Achilles tendon.

Clarithromycin (Biaxin)

Another antibiotic used in the treatment of Crohn's. As with the others there is currently little formal evidence to justify its use.

6-Mercaptopurine (6-MP, Purinethol)

6-MP is basically an oral chemotherapy drug that was found out, by accident, to be good for the treatment

167

of Crohn's disease. Like most of the anti-metabolite drugs, it interferes with the proliferation of immune system cells in the intestine, and that means they can do less damage. Immunosuppressive drugs such as 6-mercaptopurine (Purinethol) are being increasingly used for long-term treatment of Crohn's disease. They are particularly useful in the setting of a patient who is dependent on chronic high-dose steroid therapy with its severe and predictable side effects.

The medication takes approximately 3 months to take effect and some of the side effects are hair loss and low blood cell count. The hair may get really thin at first and once your body gets used to the medication, it should start to grow back. Since this series of medication can cause a form of leukemia, blood tests should be done regularly not exceeding every 3 months.

Azathioprine (Imuran)

Azathioprine is a drug that was originally used to prevent rejection in organ transplant patients. 6-MP is one of the metabolites of Azathioprine; that means that Azathioprine is converted into 6-MP in the body.

Both of these drugs have shown some degree of effectiveness when used in combination with Prednisone. Because they facilitate the use of lower steroid doses they are frequently called "steroid sparing" drugs. Most people can tolerate these drugs without difficulty thus helping avoid long term high dose steroids and the predictable associated side effects. At this time it is the consensus of experts in the field of managing Crohn's disease that it is clearly preferable to treat a patient with long term Azathioprine or 6-MP rather than with continued or even intermittent high dose steroids.

Despite impressive data from clinical trials supporting the use of 6-MP and Azathioprine in both Crohn's and ulcerative colitis, many patients are still treated with Prednisone for longer periods than are appropriate because of the erroneous perception that Azathioprine and 6-MP are more hazardous. This perception results in part from the side effect profile seen when these drugs were originally used in preventing transplant rejection and also in the treatment of leukemia. The important difference is that significantly higher doses were used in these situations than are now used in the treatment of Crohn's and ulcerative colitis. These drugs were developed in the 1950s and were first used for treating IBD some 30 years ago. Obviously a tremendous learning curve has been experienced about how to use these medications to maximize their advantages over that time period.

The minimum time to respond to the drug is approximately 3 months, however; response time can take as long as 12 months. These drugs are effective in maintaining remission in 60 - 80% of patients.

An important side effect that occurs in 3 - 5% of patients is pancreatitis. This usually occurs within a few weeks of starting treatment and is manifested by upper abdominal pain, which may radiate to the back and be associated with nausea and vomiting. If pancreatitis occurs then the patient cannot take either Azathioprine or 6-MP in the future.

Occasionally there are problems with a reduced white blood cell count. From that, it is recommended that patients have complete blood counts on a regular basis. Having blood counts performed every three months is recommended though they should be more frequent during the first few months of therapy.

The issue of how long these drugs can safely be used for has not been definitively resolved. An increasing number of patients have been maintained on these drugs for several years without any significant long-term side effects noted.

Cholestyramine / Questran ™

The most common side effect of cholestyramine use is constipation. It usually is mild but can produce fecal impaction and it can also worsen preexisting constipation and aggravate hemmorroids. Every effort should be made to avoid constipation and the best way to accomplish this is by drinking plenty of water. Other gastrointestinal side effects include cholelithiasis, pancreatitis, gastrointestinal tract bleeding, peptic ulcer, steatorrhea, anorexia, malabsorption syndrome, distention, bloating, flatulence, which is intestinal gas, nausea / vomiting, and diarrhea.

Chronic use can cause bleeding and hyperchloremic acidosis could occur, particularly in smaller patients or children. Cholestyramine is also contraindicated in patients with primary biliary cirrhosis because it can further raise serum cholesterol. Cholestyramine is relatively contraindicated treatment, which simply means that the treatment would involve a greater than normal risk to the patient's condition and would therefore not recommended, especially in patients with coronary artery disease or hemorrhoids because constipation can aggravate these conditions.

Cholestyramine absorbs and combines with bile acids, which increases removal of cholesterol. It lowers blood fats and cholesterol for patients who are at risk of getting heart disease or a stroke and is prescribed only for patients whose cholesterol level is not being controlled by diet. It is not a cure for high cholesterol. This drug also helps to relieve itching in patients with liver disease. Generic cholestyramine tablets are not yet available.

Your doctor, dentist, or pharmacist must know if any of the following conditions exist before you take cholestyramine:

Bleeding problems or blood vessel disease, constipation, gall bladder disease, hemorrhoids, kidney disease, phenylketonuria, under active thyroid, an unusual or allergic reaction to cholestyramine, other medications, foods, dyes, or preservatives; or if you are pregnant or trying to get pregnant or are breastfeeding.

Ccholestyramine tablets are taken orally. It is very important that you follow the directions on the prescription label. **Special precautions should be taken when administering this drug to children.** Under no circumstances should this medicine be given to children under 6 years of age.

Other medicines that can have adverse interactions with cholestyramine are:

Heart medicines such as digoxin or digitoxin, methotrexate penicillin G, phytonadione, propranolol, tetracycline, antibiotics, thyroid hormones, vitamin A, vitamin D, warfarin, and water pills.

Make sure you tell your doctor, dentist or pharmacist about all other medicines you are taking, including non-prescription medicines. You should also let them know if you are a frequent user of drinks with caffeine, alcohol, if you smoke or if you use illegal drugs.

These reactions to the medication may affect the way the medicine works. Check before stopping or starting any of your current medications.

Specific Medications that worsen the *symptoms* of Crohn's disease:

Non-steroidal anti-inflammatory drugs, antibiotics such as penicillin and clindamycin, antacids containing magnesium, quinidine, gold compounds, and isotretinoin (used to treat acne).

Although these drugs may worsen some of the *symptoms* of Crohn's disease, they do not appear to worsen the Crohn's *disease* itself. Always check with your doctor before taking these or any other medications.

Chapter 11

Disease Maintenance

Maintenance of Crohn's disease is an on-going, never-ending ordeal. Several areas of general bodily health are required to lead a normal, symptom free life. Depending on your individual case, symptoms, relapses and body, your maintenance efforts may assume more or less of these methods. Check with your doctor before beginning or altering any of the current methods that you use to maintain remission.

Diet and Nutrition

Good nutrition is essential in any chronic disease but especially in this illness. Because Crohn's is characterized by reduced appetite, poor absorption, and diarrhea, all of which rob the body of fluids, nutrients, vitamins, and minerals; restoration and maintenance of proper nutrition is a vital part of the personal management of the disease.

Dietary changes have been shown to positively affect the symptoms related to Crohn's disease. Although food appears to play no role in causing the disease, soft, bland foods may cause less discomfort than spicy or high-fiber foods when the disease is active. Except for restricting milk in lactose intolerant patients, most Gastroenterologists try to be flexible in planning the diets of their Crohn's patients.

Since fiber is poorly digestible, it can intensify symptoms of partial bowel obstruction; therefore, a low fiber diet may be recommended. Those patients with the disease in the small bowel are exceptionally good candidates for low fiber diets. A liquid diet may be of benefit when symptoms are more severe. When it is felt that total bowel rest is necessary, intravenous nutrition or total peripheral nutrition (TPN) may be utilized. Since poor absorption of Calcium, Folate and Vitamin B12 is predominate in patients with Crohn's, supplements for these nutrients may be helpful. The use of anti-diarrhea medications and anti-spasmodic medications can also help relieve symptoms of diarrhea and cramps.

Exercise

You should exercise 3 - 5 times a week. Exercise may include cardiovascular workouts, weight lifting, playing basketball, tennis, or some other high activity sport or just plain old walking.

Before you start any exercise program, make sure that you talk to your doctor about the program, what you intend to get out of it, and how long to give yourself to get where you want to be.

One last thought on exercise is that it is easy to make excuses to not exercise ... been there, done that. My favorites were bathroom problems, not feeling good, too tired, no energy and the best and one of my all time most used ... no time.

You must force yourself to participate in some type of activity to keep your muscles active, your bones healthy, and to help keep your heart in good health.

Laxatives

Most people with Crohn's disease do not need laxatives. However for those who have made lifestyle changes and are still constipated, doctors may recommend laxatives or enemas for a limited time. These treatments can help re-train a chronically sluggish bowel. For children, short-term treatment with laxatives, along with retraining to establish regular bowel habits, also helps prevent constipation.

Your doctor should determine when you need a laxative and which form is best. Laxatives taken by mouth are available in liquid, tablet, gum, powder, and granule forms. They work in various ways.

Bulk-forming laxatives generally are considered the safest but can interfere with absorption of some medicines. These laxatives, also known as fiber supplements, are taken with water. They absorb water in the intestine and make the stool softer. Brand names include Metamucil®, Fiber-Con®, Citrucel®, Konsyl®, and Serutan®.

Stimulants cause rhythmic muscle contractions in the intestines. Brand names include Correctol®, Dulcolax®, Purge®, Feen-A-Mint®, and Senokot®. Studies suggest that phenolphthalein, an ingredient in some stimulant laxatives, might increase a person's risk for cancer. The Food and Drug Administration has proposed a ban on all over-the-counter products containing phenolphthalein. Most laxative makers have replaced or plan to replace phenolphthalein with a safer ingredient.

Stool softeners provide moisture to the stool and prevent dehydration. These laxatives are often recommended after childbirth or surgery. Brand names include Colace®, Dialose®, and Surfak®.

Lubricants grease the stool enabling it to move through the intestine more easily. Mineral oil is the most common lubricant.

175

Saline laxatives act like a sponge to draw water into the colon for easier passage of stool. This group includes Milk of Magnesia®, Citrate of Magnesia®, and Haley's M-O®.

People who are dependent on laxatives should make every attempt to stop using them. Your doctor can assist you in this process. When the laxative is stopped, in most people, it will restore the colon's natural ability to function.

Emotional Stress

It has long since been proven that the body and mind are closely interrelated in numerous and complex ways. To that end, emotional stress can influence the course of Crohn's disease, or any other illness. High stress situations and / or acute emotional problems occasionally precede the onset or recurrence of Crohn's. Some scientists believe however that this correlation does not imply cause and effect.

Individuals with Crohn's should receive understanding and emotional support from their families and from their doctors. Some patients are helped considerably by a therapist knowledgeable about inflammatory bowel disease or about chronic illness in general. There are local support groups to help patients and their families cope with Crohn's disease.

Dealing with Relapses

The best way to deal with a relapse of Crohn's disease is to seek effective medical treatment as soon as possible. Anti-inflammatory drugs usually can handle most relapses. Your doctor and you will decide which medications are best for your particular condition.

Dealing with Attacks of Gas, Diarrhea or Pain in a Public Setting

Whenever you are away from home, plan your outing in accordance with your body's schedule. Make sure that you know where the rest rooms are located at in restaurants, shopping malls, on a trip or while using public transportation. In case of an accident, (and they happen) always carry extra underclothing or toilet tissue. Always look for a way to get by your self in short order.

Be very up front when about your needs and attacks of pain and gas. If you are not up front with yourself, you will not be able to help yourself and gain cooperation from others. Sometimes, you will need others to follow your lead and understand your situation.

Your family and close friends are aware that your condition causes you to have severe pains that come and go. There is little they can do but allow you to handle your pain in the way that is best for you.

Emotional Impact of Youngsters

Younger age groups and teenagers tend to be more severely affected by any chronic illness than adults are. Adults have learned to cope with adversity and tend to handle the emotional turmoil of a chronic disease. Therefore, the percentages of individuals who experience emotional problems in conjunction with Crohn's disease are somewhat lower adults.

Chapter 12

Food Intake

This Chapter will show the different food groups and what I personally could and could not tolerate. Each of the items will be listed but I do not endorse nor do I recommend any of the food items listed in this Chapter. Conversely, I do not suggest that any food group is not needed for general good health, nor is it my intention to be critical of any brand name item. This is simply an informational tool to help you understand what food groups were tolerated and were not tolerated by a typical Crohnie. My diet took almost 4 years to stabilize and find out what I could and could not tolerate. I typically allowed six times of an adverse reaction before I eliminated the food or drink from my diet.

Some Nutritionists recommend that patients with Crohn's disease stay away from milk, soda pop, spicy foods, red meat and high fiber foods. My response to that way of thinking is that each person is an individual with individual symptoms, problems, side effects and tolerances. You must decide, by trial and error, what your body will and will not tolerate. I recommend using weekend day's equivalent to Friday or Saturday for your "experiments" in food tasting. If you do try something that does not agree with your system, it gives you Sunday to clear it out and get back to normal so you can go back to work on Monday.

The concept of eating nutritional foods for a Crohn's patient is a never-ending challenge. What you would think would have an adverse affect on the body does nothing. What you think would be great for the body, cause severe pain, gas, diarrhea, discomfort and nausea. Once you find what your system will and won't tolerate, stick with it. Learn how to cook those items different ways using different spices or side dishes. Eventually, you will have a diet that is healthy, nutritional and most of all, well tolerated.

The strongest recommendation I can make to any Crohnie is not to let others decide what it is you eat and don't eat. It is your body and you are going to deal with the results of what you ingest. If you let somebody talk you into a steak, and you know before you eat that steak that you don't tolerate steak well, then get ready to pay the price ... BY YOURSELF ... because no one will be around when you have to "pay the fiddler" (sort of speak). Eat what you feel comfortable eating. If there is a steak fry and you don't tolerate steak well, bring a piece of chicken. Don't eat something that is going to be rough on you "just to fit it" because it is simply not worth it. Most of your friends and family have no clue how you feel after eating something that doesn't set well with the body.

Always keep in mind that it is YOU who are going to both enjoy your meal and be satisfied, or eat your meal and be miserable.

The most important thing to remember: *Take everything in moderation.*

The Basic Food Groups

"It has been said that if you eat the correct amount of servings in the correct portions from the 4 major food groups that you will always be eating "right". If you definitely don't want to put yourself on any sort of strict diet, then at least try to follow these rules and you should

179

shed some pounds. If you're watching calories as well, turn the page to our Calorie Counter. If you're in search of recipes check out our recipe link. Oh-you'll notice that we haven't included fats, sweets or alcohol in our food groups. As hard as we tried, we couldn't find any source that considered these useful foods so our only advice is use them sparingly." *Better Homes and Gardens NEW COOKBOOK (Copyright 1989)*

Vegetables and Fruits

Foods in this Group - All vegetables and fruits (fresh, canned, frozen or dried) and their juices.

Major Nutrients - Carbohydrates, fiber and vitamins A and C. Dark green vegetables are good sources of ribloflavin, folacin, iron and magnesium.

Breads and Cereals

Foods in this Group - All foods based on whole grains or enriched flour or meal. Includes breads, biscuits, muffins, waffles, pancakes, pasta, rice and cereals.

Major Nutrients - Carbohydrates, protein, thiamine, riboflavin, niacin B vitamins and iron. Whole-grain products provide magnesium, fiber and folacin.

Milk and Cheese

Foods in this Group - All types of milk, yogurt, cheese, ice milk, ice cream and foods prepared with milk (milk shakes, puddings, and creamed soups.)

Major Nutrients - Protein, calcium, riboflavin and vitamins A, B6 and B12. When fortified, these products also provide Vitamin D.

Meats, Fish, Poultry and Beans

Foods in this Group - Beef, veal, lamb, pork, poultry, fish, shellfish, dry beans or peas, soybeans, lentils, eggs, peanuts and other nuts, peanut butter and seeds.

Major Nutrients - Protein, phosphorus and vitamin B6. Foods of animal origin provide vitamin B12. Meats, dry beans and dry peas provide iron. Liver and egg yolks provide vitamin A.

Well Tolerated Food and Drink

Fruits and Vegetables

Apricots, asparagus, bananas, blackberries, blueberries, boysenberries, broccoli, cantaloupe, carrots, celery, cherries, cranberries, cucumbers, garlic, green onions, honeydew, kiwifruit, mangoes, mushrooms, nectarines, onions, papayas, peaches, pears, pickles, pineapple, plums, pomegranates, potatoes, raspberries, strawberries, watermelon, all fruit juices except cranberry juice and tomato juice.

Dairy Products

Bleu cheese, brie, butter, cottage cheese, cheddar cheese, cream cheese, jack cheese, 2% milk, parmesian cheese, skim milk, sour cream, Swiss cheese, whipping cream, yogurt.

Meat, Poultry and Fish

Bacon, catfish, chicken, cod, eggs, ham, mussels, oysters, salmon, sausage, shrimps, tuna, turkey.

Breads

Bagels, biscuits, bread (wheat, white, 7 grain, 9 grain, 12 grain, dark rye, white rye, sourdough), dinner rolls, rice.

*Soft Drinks / Alcohol**

All Coke, Pepsi and Generic soda products; Stolychania®, Jim Beam®, Gordon's® Vodka, Parrot Bay®, Absolut®, SKYY®, Canadian Club®, Canadian Mist®, Seagrams 7®, Christian Brothers®.

*(Alcohol intake is closely monitored and regulated, in other words, I don't drink a lot, but I do have an adult beverage now and then. These are the alcohol beverages that I have consumed, in moderation, which did not have had an affect on my Crohn's such as cramps, headache or diarrhea.).

Not Well Tolerated Food and Drink

Fruits and Vegetables

Apples, bell peppers, cabbage, corn, grapefruit, grapes, jalapenos, lemons, lettuce, limes, oranges, peas, peppers, prunes, raisins, sauerkraut, snow peas, tangerines, tangelos, tomatoes, cranberry juice, tomato juice, tomato sauce, tomato paste.

Dairy Products

Acidophilus milk, chocolate milk, cream (half and half), margarine, whole milk.

Meat, Poultry and Fish

Crab, lobster, all shellfish, steak, all red meat, spicy meats, any fried foods.

Breads

Donuts, muffins, nuts of any kind.

Soft Drinks / Alcohol*

Any beer, gin, tequila, wine, wine coolers, generic vodka or rum.

*(Alcohol intake is closely monitored and regulated, in other words, I don't drink a lot, but I do have an adult beverage now and then. These are the alcohol beverages that I have consumed, in moderation, which did have an affect on my Crohn's such as cramps, headache or diarrhea).

Daily Supplements

I take the following supplements every day. In order to make sure that my system is not thrown out of whack by the combination of these supplements, I take a portion of them in the morning at about 6:00 am. The balance of these supplements is taken in the afternoon between 1:00 pm and 1:30 pm.

This combination of vitamins and supplements has worked for me in keeping my Crohn's under control as well as helping me with my daily dietary needs to support my nutritional needs as well as my exercise program. These supplements may or may not work for you under your circumstances.

My suggestion is to consult your doctor and use a "trial and error" method to find out what works for you. This regiment of supplements and food tolerances took several years for me to develop and get a balance that would work for my body:

Morning:

Allopurinol (when needed), Bayer Aspirin®, Benadryl®, Chlortabs, Flax Seed Oil, Metamucil®, Pentasa (when needed) and Vitamin E

Afternoon:

Fish oil, Vitamin B1, Vitamin C, Calcium, Protein drink with milk, and Milk Thistle

Chapter 13

Medication Side Effect Index

All the medications listed here may be either prescribed for Irritable Bowel Syndrome, Inflammatory Bowel Disease, the side effects caused by these diseases or they also may be being used in clinical trials for these conditions. Most of the common and rare side effects are listed along with withdrawal and overdose symptoms where appropriate.

Other side effects not listed in this Index may occur in some patients. If you notice any other side effect, check with your doctor immediately. This information should only be used as a guideline to understand how different medications may affect you. Always consult your doctor or your pharmacist for complete information about the prescription medications that you are given. If you are pregnant, breastfeeding or thinking of becoming pregnant, check with your doctor before taking any medications.

This Chapter has space for you to take notes regarding side effects you experience. Don't be afraid to use this area to make notes to your self. Remember that everybody is different and will experience different side effects, and as I previously said, some of those side effects may not be listed here.

Several of the medications listed in this section will cause a condition known as *Cushing's syndrome*. Symptoms of Cushing's syndrome may include acne, depression, excessive hair growth, high blood pressure, humped upper back, insomnia, moon-faced appearance, muscle weakness, obese trunk, paranoia, stretch marks, stunted growth in children, susceptibility to bruising, fractures, infections and wasted limbs. Cushing's syndrome may also trigger diabetes mellitus.

If it is left uncorrected, Cushing's syndrome may become serious and you should pay special attention to any of the symptoms of this condition and if any symptoms are noticed, notify your doctor immediately.

For more medication information, visit www.healthsqr.com. I have found that they have the most complete and up-to-date medication information available.

Index of Medications

6-MP (Mercaptopurine, Purinethol)

AcipHex (Rabeprazole sodium)
Aclovate (Alclometasone dipropionate)
Actigall (Ursodiol / Urso)
Antacids (Brand names: Gaviscon,
    Maalox, ylanta, Rolaids, Tums)
Arava (Leflunomide)
Axid
Azathioprine (Imuran)
Azulfadine (Sulfasalazine)

Carafate (Sucralfate)
Cell Cept (Mycophenolate)
Cholestyramine
Chronulac Syrup (Lactulose)
Ciprofloxacin (Cipro)

Colace (Docusate, Ex-Lax Stool Softener,
    Phillips' Liqui-Gels, Surfak Liqui-Gels)
Colazal (Balsalazide disodium)
Compazine (Prochlorperazine)
Cyclocort (Amcinonide)
Cyclosporin
Cytotec (Misoprostol)

Dapsone
Decadron Tablets (Dexamethasone)
Dicyclomine hydrochloride (Bentyl)
Dilaudid (Hydromorphone hydrochloride)
Dipentum (Olsalazine sodium)

Donnatal (Phenobarbital, Hyoscyamine
  sulfate,
Atropine sulfate, Scopolamine hydrobromide,
Bellatal

Elocon (Mometasone furoate)
Enbrel (Etanercept)
Entocort
Erythromycin, Oral (E.E.S., E-Mycin,
  ERYC, Ery-Tab, Erythrocin, PCE)

Flagyl (Metronidazole)
Fosamax (Alendronate sodium)

Helidac Therapy (Bismuth subsalicylate,
Metronidazole, Tetracycline hydrochloride)
Hydrocortisone Skin Preparations (Cetacort,
Hytone, Nutracort)

Imodium (Loperamide hydrochloride)
Infliximab (Remicade)

Levsin (Hycoscyamine sulfate, Anaspaz,
Levbid, Levsinex)
Librax
Lidex (Fluocinonide)
Lomotil (Diphenoxylate hydrochloride, Atropine
sulfate)
Lopid (Gemfibrozil)

Medrol (Methylprednisolone)
Methotrexate (Rheumatrex)

Nexium (Esomeprazole magnesium)

Oprelvekin (Interleukin-11, recombinant,

rIL-11)
Oral Mesalamine (Asacol, Pentasa, Mesasal,
Salofalk)

Pancrease (Pancrelipase, Creon, Pancrease MT,
    Viokase, Ultrase)
Pepcid (Famotidine, Pepcid AC, Pepcid RPD)
Prednisone
Prevacid (Lansoprazole)
Prilosec (Omeprazole
Psorcon (Diflorasone diacetate)

Rectal Mesalamine (Rowasa, Salofalk)
Reglan (Metoclopramide hydrochloride)

Temovate (Clobetasol propionate,
    Cormax)
Tetracycline (Achromycin V, Sumycin)
Thalidomide (Thalomid)
Topicort (Desoximetasone)
Tridesilon (Desonide, DesOwen)

Zantac
Zyloprim (Allopurinol)

6-MP (Mercaptopurine, Purinethol)

Check with your Doctor if any of the following side effects appear:

Darkening of skin, diarrhea, headache, skin rash and itching, weakness.

Always notify your Doctor if any of the following side effects appear:

Unusual tiredness or weakness, yellow eyes or skin, joint pain, loss of appetite, nausea and vomiting, swelling of feet or lower legs, sores in mouth and on lips.

Immediately notify your Doctor if any of the following side effects appear:

Black tarry stools, blood in urine or stools, cough or hoarseness, fever or chills, lower back or side pain, painful or difficult urination, pinpoint red spots on skin, unusual bleeding or bruising.

Toxicity and adverse reactions:

Because of the way cancer medicine act on the body, there is a chance that they might cause other unwanted effects months or years after the medicine is used. These delayed effects may include certain types of cancer which should be discussed with your doctor.

Mercaptopurine may still produce side effects after you stopped treatment. During this period of time, check with your doctor if you notice any of the following side effects:

Black tarry stools, blood in urine or stools, cough or hoarseness, fever or chills, lower back or side pain, painful or difficult urination, pinpoint red spots on skin, unusual bleeding or bruising.

AcipHex (Rabeprazole sodium)

Check with your Doctor if any of the following side effects appear:

Absence of breathing, agitation, amnesia, bile duct inflammation, breast enlargement, confusion, deafness, dry skin, eye pain, fluid retention of the face, hangover effect, headache, heavy periods, hyperactivity, salivary gland enlargement, shingles, skin discoloration or scaling, slowed breathing, thirst, twitching, urinary incontinence, vaginal discharge, vein inflammation, visual disturbance.

Always notify your Doctor if any of the following side effects appear:

Abdominal pain, abnormal dreams, abnormal stools, abnormal vision, allergic reaction, anxiety, arthritis, asthma, belching, bladder inflammation, bone pain, bruising, bursitis, cataract, chills, constipation, decreased sex drive, dehydration, depression, diarrhea, difficult breathing, difficult periods, dry eyes, dry mouth, ear infection, fainting, fatigue, fever, fluid retention, frequent urination, gas, glaucoma, gout, gum inflammation, hair loss, heart attack, hiccup, high blood pressure, hives, hyperventilation, increased appetite, inflammation of

191

the esophagus, inflammation of the pancreas, insomnia, irregular heartbeat, itching, laryngitis, leg cramps, loss of appetite, migraine, mouth inflammation, mouth sores, muscle pain, nausea, nerve pain, nervous system disorder, nervousness, overactive thyroid, painful urination, pins and needles sensation, pounding heartbeat, rash, rectal bleeding or inflammation, ringing in the ears, sensitivity to sunlight, sleepiness, slowed or racing heartbeat, stiff neck, stiffness, stomach upset or inflammation, sweating, tongue inflammation, tremor, vertigo, vomiting, weakness, weight gain or loss.

Immediately notify your Doctor if any of the following side effects appear:

Abdominal swelling, blood clot, blood in the urine, blood vessel enlargement, bloody diarrhea, chest pain, convulsion, dizziness, gallbladder disease, impotence, inflammation of the small intestine, intestinal bleeding, irregular heartbeat, kidney stone, liver disorders, nervous disorders, nosebleed, stomach bleeding, testicular inflammation, under active thyroid.

Toxicity and adverse reactions:

If you have stomach ulcers caused by the *H. pylori* bacteria, AcipHex could make the condition slightly worse. Your Doctor may order a test for *H. pylori* before prescribing this drug.

It is especially important to check with your doctor before combining AcipHex with the following medications: Cyclosporine (Neoral, Sandimmune), Ketoconazole (Nizoral), Digoxin (Lanoxin).

Aclovate (Alclometasone dipropionate)

Check with your Doctor if any of the following side effects appear:

Acne-like pimples, allergic rash/inflammation, burning, dryness, infection, irritation, itching, pale spots, prickly heat, rash, redness, stretch marks on skin.

Always notify your Doctor if any of the following side effects appear:

If you have any other allergic reaction to the drug.

Immediately notify your Doctor if any of the following side effects appear:

In a child, an overdose of Aclovate may cause increased pressure within the skull leading to bulging soft spots in an infant's head or headache.

Toxicity and adverse reactions:

For areas of deep-seated, persistent rash, your Doctor may recommend a thick layer of Aclovate cream or ointment topped with waterproof bandaging. Do not use bandaging unless your Doctor advises you to.

Aclovate is for use only on the skin so be very careful to keep it out of your eyes and avoid using the product on your face, underarms, or groin, unless your Doctor tells you to. Do not use Aclovate to treat diaper rash or apply it in the diaper area.

If you use Aclovate over large areas of skin for prolonged periods of time, the amount of hormone absorbed into your bloodstream may eventually lead to Cushing's syndrome. The drug should not be used on children under 1 year of age or for more than 3 weeks in children older than 1 year.

Check with your Doctor before combining Aclovate with other more potent steroids, since this could lead to undesirably large amounts of hormone circulating in your bloodstream.

Drug absorbed from Aclovate cream or ointment into the bloodstream may find its way into an unborn child's blood, or may seep into breast milk. To avoid any possible harm to your child, use Aclovate very sparingly, and only with your Doctor's permission.

Actigall (Ursodiol / Urso)

Check with your Doctor if any of the following side effects appear:

Abdominal pain, allergy, arthritis, back pain, bronchitis.

Always notify your Doctor if any of the following side effects appear:

Cough, diarrhea, dizziness, fatigue, flu-like symptoms, gas, hair loss, headache, high blood sugar, indigestion, insomnia, joint pain, menstrual
194

pain, muscle and bone pain, nasal inflammation, nausea.

Immediately notify your Doctor if any of the following side effects appear:

Chest pain, constipation, sinus inflammation, skin rash, sore throat, stomach or intestinal disorder, stomach ulcer, upper respiratory tract infection, urinary tract infection, viral infection, vomiting.

Toxicity and adverse reactions:

Under the brand name Urso, its active ingredient is prescribed to treat liver disease caused by hardening and blockage of the bile ducts known as primary biliary cirrhosis.

Actigall is not a quick remedy and it takes months of Actigall therapy to dissolve gallstones. There is also a possibility of incomplete dissolution and recurrence of stones. Your Doctor will weigh Actigall against alternative treatments and recommend the best one for you. Actigall is most effective if your gallstones are small or floatable, which means high in cholesterol. Most importantly, your gallbladder must still be functioning properly.

Take Actigall exactly as prescribed or the gallstones may dissolve too slowly or not dissolve at all. During treatment, your Doctor will do periodic ultrasound exams to see if your stones are dissolving.

Although Actigall is not known to cause liver damage, it is theoretically possible in some people.

Your Doctor may run blood tests for liver function before you start to take Actigall and again while you are taking it.

It is especially important to check with your Doctor before combining Actigall with Aluminum-based antacid medications such as Alu-Cap, Alu-Tab, and Rolaids; Cholesterol-lowering medications, such as Atromid-S, Lopid, Mevacor, Questran, and Colestid; Estrogens such as Premarin and any Oral contraceptives

Antacids (Brand names: Gaviscon, Maalox, Mylanta, Rolaids, Tums)

Check with your Doctor if any of the following side effects appear:

Chalky taste, constipation, diarrhea, increased thirst, stomach cramps.

The following symptoms are symptoms of an overdose. Notify your Doctor immediately:

For aluminum-containing antacids (Gaviscon, Maalox, Mylanta)

Bone pain, constipation (severe and continuing), feeling of discomfort (continuing), loss of appetite (continuing), mood or mental changes, muscle weakness, swelling of wrists or ankles, weight loss (unusual).

For calcium-containing antacids (Mylanta, Rolaids, Tums)

196

Constipation (severe and continuing), difficult or painful urination, frequent urge to urinate, headache (continuing), loss of appetite (continuing), mood or mental changes, muscle pain or twitching, nausea or vomiting, nervousness or restlessness, slow breathing, unpleasant taste, unusual tiredness or weakness.

For magnesium-containing antacids (Gaviscon, Maalox, Mylanta)

Difficult or painful urination, dizziness or lightheadedness, irregular heartbeat, mood or mental changes, unusual tiredness or weakness.

Toxicity and adverse reactions:

Do not take antacids for longer than 2 weeks or in larger than recommended doses unless directed by your Doctor. If your symptoms persist, contact Doctor immediately.

Antacids should be used only for occasional relief of stomach upset.

Do not take antacids if you have signs of appendicitis or an inflamed bowel. These symptoms include stomach or lower abdominal pain, cramping, bloating, soreness, nausea, or vomiting.

If you are sensitive to or have ever had an allergic reaction to aluminum, calcium, magnesium, or simethicone, do not take an antacid containing these ingredients. If you are elderly and have bone problems or if you are taking care of an elderly person with Alzheimer's disease, do not use an antacid containing aluminum.

If you are taking any prescription drug, check with your Doctor before you take an antacid.

If you have kidney disease, do not take an antacid containing aluminum or magnesium. If you are on a sodium-restricted diet, do not take Gaviscon without checking first with your Doctor.

It is especially important to check with your Doctor before combining antacids with Cellulose sodium phosphate (Calcibind), Isoniazid (Rifamate), Ketoconazole (Nizoral), Mecamylamine (Inversine), Methenamine (Mandelamine), Sodium polystyrene sulfonate resin (Kayexalate) or Tetracycline antibiotics (Achromycin, Minocin).

Arava (Leflunomide)

Check with your Doctor if any of the following side effects appear:

Abdominal pain, back pain, bronchitis, cough, diarrhea, dizziness, hair loss, headache, high blood pressure, indigestion, itching, joint disorders, loss of appetite, mouth ulcers, nausea, rash, respiratory infection, sore throat, stomach inflammation, tendon inflammation, urinary tract infection, vomiting, weakness, weight loss.

Always notify your Doctor if any of the following side effects appear:

Abscess, acne, anxiety, bruising, bursitis, cataracts, chest pain, colitis, conjunctivitis, dermatitis, diabetes, difficulty breathing, dry mouth, dry skin, eczema, eye problems, fever, flu-like symptoms, frequent urination, gas, general feeling of illness, gingivitis, hair discoloration, hernia, herpes infection, hyperthyroidism, insomnia, joint pain and inflammation, leg cramps, muscle aches, muscle cramps, nail disorders, skin bumps, pain, purple spots on skin, skin discoloration, skin tingling, sleep disorders, sweating, swelling, tarry stools, taste problems, tooth problems, vaginal fungal infection, varicose veins, vertigo.

Immediately notify your Doctor if any of the following side effects appear:

Allergic reaction, anemia, angina, asthma, blood in the urine, blurred vision, bone pain, constipation, cysts, depression, fungal infection of the mouth, fungal infection of the skin, gallstones, lung problems, menstrual disorders, migraine, mouth and throat inflammation, nasal inflammation, neck pain, nosebleeds, prostate disorder, rapid heartbeat, sinus inflammation, painful urination, palpitations, pelvic pain, pneumonia, skin ulcers.

Toxicity and adverse reactions:

You MUST NOT take Arava if you are pregnant as it can harm the developing baby. If you are still in your childbearing years, your Doctor will want to see negative results from a pregnancy test before starting you on Arava. You will also need to use reliable contraceptive measures as long as you take the medication.

If you become pregnant while taking Arava, your Doctor should stop the medication immediately and prescribe a regimen of Questran in 8-gram doses 3 times a day for 11 days. Questran helps to clear Arava from the bloodstream, possibly preventing harm to the unborn child.

Arava is potentially damaging to the liver. Your Doctor should test your liver function before starting Arava therapy, and will conduct monthly blood tests for a while after therapy begins. If you have significant liver disease, including hepatitis, you'll be unable to take Arava. If you develop liver problems while taking the medication, your dose will have to be reduced or eliminated.

Theoretically, Arava may interfere with the body's ability to fight off infection. This medication is therefore not recommended for people with cancer, bone marrow problems, severe infections, AIDS, or any other immune system problems. You should also avoid immunization with live vaccines while taking Arava.

Poor kidney function can increase the amount of Arava in your system. Your Doctor should prescribe the medication cautiously if you're subject to kidney problems.

Arava does not appear to cause fetal harm when taken by the father prior to conception. Nevertheless, if you plan to father a child, your Doctor will instruct you to stop taking Arava and will prescribe a regimen of Questran to clear Arava from your system.

It is especially important to check with your Doctor before combining Arava with Cholestyramine (Prevalite, Questran), Methotrexate (Rheumatrex), Advil, Aleve, Motrin, and Naprosyn, Rifampin (Rifadin, Rifamate, Rifater) or Tolbutamide (Orinase).

Axid

Check with your Doctor if any of the following side effects appear:

Abdominal pain, diarrhea, dizziness, gas, headache, indigestion, inflammation of the nose, nausea, pain, sore throat, vomiting, weakness.

Always notify your Doctor if any of the following side effects appear:

Abnormal dreams, anxiety, back pain, dry mouth, fever, and inability to sleep, muscle pain, nervousness, rash, and sleepiness.

Immediately notify your Doctor if any of the following side effects appear:

Chest pain, constipation, dimmed vision, increased cough, infection, itching, loss of appetite, stomach/intestinal problems, tooth problems.

Toxicity and adverse reactions:

If you are sensitive to or have ever had an allergic reaction to Axid or similar drugs such as Zantac, you should not take this medication. Make sure your

Doctor is aware of any drug reactions you have experienced.

Axid could mask a stomach malignancy so if you continue to have any problems, notify your Doctor immediately. If you have moderate to severe kidney disease, your Doctor will reduce your dosage.

It is especially important to check with your doctor before combining Axid with aspirin, especially in high doses.

Azathioprine (Imuran)

Check with your Doctor if any of the following side effects appear:

Loss of appetite, nausea or vomiting, skin rash.

Always notify your Doctor if any of the following side effects appear:

Cough or hoarseness, fever or chills, lower back or side pain, painful or difficult urination, unusual tiredness or weakness, black tarry stools, blood in urine or stools, pinpoint red spots on skin, unusual bleeding or bruising, fast heartbeat, sudden fever, muscle or joint pain, nausea, vomiting, severe diarrhea, redness or blisters on skin, shortness of breath, sores in mouth and on lips, stomach pain, swelling of feet or lower legs, unusual feeling of discomfort or sudden illness.

Toxicity and adverse reactions:

Your doctor will watch for liver problems, which this medicine may cause. Because of the way this medicine acts on the body, there is a chance that it might cause other unwanted effects that may not occur until months or years after the medicine is used. These delayed effects may include certain types of cancer, such as leukemia, lymphoma, or skin cancer. The risk of cancer seems to be lower in people taking Azathioprine for arthritis, and you should discuss these possible effects with your doctor.

After you stop this medicine, there may still be some side effects. During this time notify your doctor as soon as possible if any of the following side effects appear:

Black tarry stools, blood in urine, cough or hoarseness, fever or chills, lower back or side pain, painful or difficult urination, pinpoint red spots on skin, unusual bleeding or bruising.

Azulfadine (Sulfasalazine)

Check with your Doctor if any of the following side effects appear:

Abdominal or stomach pain or upset, diarrhea, loss of appetite, nausea or vomiting.

Immediately notify your Doctor if any of the following side effects appear:

Aching of joints, continuing headache, itching, increased sensitivity of skin to sunlight, skin rash, aching of joints and muscles, back, leg, or stomach

203

pains, bloody diarrhea, bluish fingernails, lips, or skin; chest pain, cough, difficult breathing, difficulty in swallowing, fever, chills, or sore throat, general feeling of discomfort or illness, loss of appetite, pale skin, redness, blistering, peeling, or loosening of skin, unusual bleeding or bruising, unusual tiredness or weakness, yellow eyes or skin.

Toxicity and adverse reactions:

In some patients this medicine may also cause the urine or skin to become orange-yellow. This side effect does not need medical attention.

Carafate (Sucralfate)

Check with your Doctor if any of the following side effects appear:

Constipation.

Always notify your Doctor if any of the following side effects appear:

Back pain, diarrhea, dizziness, dry mouth, gas, headache, indigestion, insomnia, itching, nausea, sleepiness, stomach upset, vertigo, vomiting.

Immediately notify your Doctor if any of the following side effects appear:

Allergic reactions such as hives, breathing difficulty or rash.

The following symptoms are symptoms of an overdose. Notify your Doctor immediately:

Abdominal pain, indigestion, nausea, vomiting.

Toxicity and adverse reactions:

Carafate works best when taken on an empty stomach. If you take an antacid to relieve pain, avoid doing it within one-half hour before or after you take Carafate.

If you have kidney failure or are on dialysis, your Doctor will be cautious about prescribing this medication. Use of Carafate while taking aluminum-containing antacids may increase the possibility of aluminum poisoning in those with kidney failure.

It is especially important to check with your Doctor before combining Carafate with antacids such as Mylanta and Maalox; Coumadin, Cimetidine (Tagamet), Digoxin (Lanoxin), Dicyclomine (Bentyl), Ketoconazole (Nizoral), Levothyroxine (Synthroid), Phenytoin (Dilantin), Quinidine (Quinidex), Quinolone antibiotics such as Ciprofloxacin (Cipro) and Floxin; Ranitidine (Zantac), Tetracycline (Sumycin) and Theophylline (Theo-Dur).

Cell Cept (Mycophenolate)

Check with your Doctor if any of the following side effects appear:

Constipation, diarrhea, headache, heartburn, nausea, stomach pain, vomiting, weakness, acne, dizziness, skin rash, trouble in sleeping.

205

Always notify your Doctor if any of the following side effects appear:

Blood in the urine, chest pain, cough or hoarseness, fever or chills, increased cough, lower back or side pain, painful or difficult urination, shortness of breath, swelling of feet or lower legs, abdominal pain, black, tarry stools, bloody vomit, enlarged gums, irregular heartbeat, joint pain, muscle pain, pinpoint red spots on the skin, red, inflamed, bleeding gums, sores inside mouth, trembling or shaking of hands or feet, unusual bleeding or bruising, white patches on the mouth, tongue, or throat.

Cholestyramine

Contact your Doctor is any of the following side effects appear:

Constipation, diarrhea, dizziness, headache, heartburn, indigestion, loss of appetite, nausea, vomiting, skin rash or irritation, including the tongue and perianal area stomach upset, belching, or bloating.

Immediately contact your Doctor if any of the following side effects appear:

Bloody or black tarry stools, unusual bleeding, severe stomach pain with nausea and vomiting, noticeable weight loss.

Toxicity and adverse reactions:

Cholestyramine can cause toxicity and / or have adverse reactions with heart medicines such as digoxin or digitoxin, methotrexate penicillin G, phytonadione, propranolol, tetracycline, antibiotics, thyroid hormones, vitamin A, vitamin D, warfarin, and water pills.

Make sure you tell your doctor, dentist or pharmacist about all other medicines you are taking, including non-prescription medicines. You should also let them know if you are a frequent user of drinks with caffeine, alcohol, if you smoke or if you use illegal drugs.

Some adverse reactions are constipation, cholelithiasis which are typically called gallstones, pancreatitis, gastrointestinal tract bleeding, peptic ulcer, steatorrhea, which is also known as gluten intolerance; anorexia, malabsorption syndrome, distention, bloating, flatulence, which is intestinal gas, nausea, vomiting, and diarrhea.

Chronulac Syrup (Lactulose)

Check with your Doctor if any of the following side effects appear:

Diarrhea, gas, intestinal cramps, nausea, potassium and fluid loss, vomiting.

The following symptoms are symptoms of an overdose. Notify your Doctor immediately:

Abdominal cramps, diarrhea.

Toxicity and adverse reactions:

207

Because of its sugar content, this medication should be used with caution if you have diabetes.

It is especially important to check with your Doctor before combining Chronulac with non-absorbable antacids such as Maalox and Mylanta.

Ciprofloxacin (Cipro)

Check with your Doctor if any of the following side effects appear:

Mild upset stomach, mild diarrhea), vomiting, stomach pain, headache, restlessness, change in sense of taste, increased sensitivity of skin to sunlight.

Always notify your Doctor if any of the following side effects appear:

Blistering of skin, sensation of skin burning, skin itching, rash, redness, or swelling, skin rash, itching, hives, difficulty breathing or swallowing, swelling of the face or throat, yellowing of the skin or eyes, dark urine, pale or dark stools, blood in urine, unusual tiredness, sunburn or blistering, seizures or convulsions, vaginal infection, vision changes, pain, inflammation, or rupture of a tendon.

Toxicity and adverse reactions:

Serious and fatal reactions have occurred when Cipro was taken in combination with theophylline (Theo-Dur). These reactions have included cardiac arrest, seizures, status epilepticus, which is a continuous attack of epilepsy with no period of consciousness, and respiratory failure.

Antacids containing magnesium and aluminum, Carafate, supplements and other products containing calcium, iron, or zinc, Videx chewable tablets and pediatric powder can interfere with the absorption of Cipro and should be taken no less than 6 hours before or 2 hours after a dose of Cipro. You should also avoid taking Cipro with milk or yogurt alone, though calcium taken as part of a full meal appears to have no significant effect on the drug.

Cipro may increase the effects of   caffeine.

It is especially important to check with your Doctor before combining Cipro and Cyclophosphamide (Cytoxan), Cyclosporine (Sandimmune, Neoral), Glyburide (DiaBeta, Glynase, Micronase), Metoprolol (Lopressor), Phenytoin (Dilantin), Probenecid (Benemid) or Coumadin.

It is important that your Doctor monitor your condition on a regular basis because continued or prolonged use of this medication may result in a growth of bacteria that do not respond to this medication which can cause a secondary infection.

Colace (Docusate, Ex-Lax Stool Softener, Phillips' Liqui-Gels, Surfak Liqui-Gels)

Check with your Doctor if any of the following side effects appear:

Abdominal pain, bitter taste, throat irritation, and nausea (mainly associated with use of the syrup and liquid), rash.

Toxicity and adverse reactions:

Colace is helpful for people who have had recent rectal surgery, people with heart problems, high blood pressure, hemorrhoids, or hernias, and women who have just had babies.

Colace is for short-term relief only, unless your Doctor directs otherwise. It usually takes a day or two for the drug to achieve its laxative effect although some people may need to wait 4 or 5 days. Sof-Lax Overnight works in 6 to 12 hours. Colace Microenema works in 2 to 15 minutes.

If you are going to use the Colace Microenema, lubricate the tip by pushing out a drop of the medication. Slowly insert the full length of the nozzle into the rectum. (Stop halfway for children aged 3 to 12 years of age.) Squeeze out the contents of the tube. Remove the nozzle before you release your grip on the tube.

Do not take this product if you are taking mineral oil. If you have noticed a change in your bowel habits that have lasted for 2 weeks, ask your Doctor before you use this product. If you bleed from the rectum or you do not have a bowel movement after using this product, stop using it and call your doctor; you may have a more serious condition. Do not use any laxative for more than a week without your Doctor's approval.

Colazal (Balsalazide disodium)

Check with your Doctor if any of the following side effects appear:

Back pain, cough, cramps, dizziness, dry mouth, fatigue, fever, flu-like disorder, frequent stools, gas, loss of appetite, muscle aches, pain, runny nose, sinus inflammation, sleeplessness, sore throat, stomach upset.

Always notify your Doctor if any of the following side effects appear:

Abdominal pain, diarrhea, headache, joint pain, nausea, and vomiting, respiratory infection.

Immediately notify your Doctor if any of the following side effects appear:

Bloody urine, constipation, rectal bleeding, urinary disorders.

Toxicity and adverse reactions:

Although there have been no reports of kidney damage from Colazal, other products containing Mesalamine are known to have caused this problem. If you have kidney disease, your Doctor will monitor your condition closely during treatment with Colazal. Some cases of fatal liver disease have been reported during treatment with Colazal. If you have a liver problem, make sure your Doctor is aware of it before you start treatment.

Do not take Colazal if you are allergic to Rowasa or salicylates such as aspirin.

If you have pyloric stenosis, which is the narrowing of the stomach outlet, Colazal capsules may be slow to pass through the digestive tract.

Although many people get significant relief from Colazal, you should be aware that in rare cases it makes the symptoms worse.

While drug interactions with Colazal have not yet been studied, it is possible that oral antibiotics could interfere with the release of this medication in the colon.

Compazine (Prochlorperazine)

Check with your Doctor if any of the following side effects appear:

Mild constipation decreased sweating, dizziness, drowsiness, dryness of mouth, nasal congestion, menstrual irregularity, decreased sex drive, photosensitivity, swelling, pain or milk secretion in breasts, weight gain.

Always notify your Doctor if any of the following side effects appear:

Blurred vision, change in color vision, fainting, loss of balance, night blindness, restlessness, stiffness in legs and arms, trembling and shaking of hands and fingers, abdominal or stomach pains, aching muscles and joints, agitation or excitement, chest pains, difficulty in sleeping / bizarre dreams, urinating dark urine, fever and chills, hair loss, headaches, hot, dry skin or lack of sweating, rash or severely itchy skin, mild confusion, nausea, vomiting, or diarrhea, prolonged, painful, inappropriate erection, redness of hands, shivering, seizures, convulsions, severe constipation, skin or eye discoloration (tan, yellow, or blue-gray), sore throat and fever, sores in mouth, severe sunburn, unusual bleeding or bruising, tiredness or weakness, muscle weakness, pain in joints.

Immediately notify your Doctor if any of the following side effects appear:

Difficulty in breathing, speaking, or swallowing, inability to move eyes, increased blinking or eyelid spasms, lip smacking or puckering, muscle spasms of face, neck, body, arms, or legs causing unusual postures or unusual facial expressions, puffing of cheeks, rapid or worm-like movements of tongue, sticking out of tongue, twitching, uncontrolled movement or twisting of mouth, neck, arms, legs, or trunk, slow or irregular heart beat, recurrent fainting.

The following are signs of neuroleptic malignant syndrome. Immediately notify your Doctor if any of these side effects appear:

Severe confusion or coma, difficulty in speaking or swallowing, difficulty in breathing, drooling, fever, irregular (high or low) blood pressure, increased sweating, loss of bladder control, severe muscle stiffness, severe trembling or shaking, rapid heartbeat.

213

Cyclocort (Amcinonide)

Check with your Doctor if any of the following side effects appear:

Dryness, excessive growth of hair, infection, inflammation of hair follicles, inflammation of the skin around the mouth, irritation, prickly heat, skin eruptions resembling acne, softening of the skin, stretch marks.

Always notify your Doctor if any of the following side effects appear:

Burning, itching, soreness, stinging sensation.

Toxicity and adverse reactions:

When you use Cyclocort, you will inevitably absorb some of the medication through your skin and into the bloodstream. Too much absorption can lead to unwanted side effects elsewhere in the body so in order to keep this problem to a minimum, avoid using large amounts of Cyclocort over large areas, and do not cover it with airtight dressings such as plastic wrap or adhesive bandages unless specifically told to by your Doctor.

If you are sensitive to or have ever had an allergic reaction to Amcinonide or other steroid medications, you should not use Cyclocort. Make sure your Doctor is aware of any drug reactions you have experienced.

Cyclosporin

Check with your Doctor if any of the following side effects appear:

Increase in hair growth, trembling and shaking of hands, acne or oily skin, headache, leg cramps, nausea.

The following side effects must be monitored closely by your Doctor:

High blood pressure, kidney problems, liver problems, changes in blood chemistry

Always notify your Doctor if any of the following side effects appear:

Bleeding, tender, or enlarged gums, convulsions, seizures, fever or chills, frequent urge to urinate, vomiting, confusion, general feeling of discomfort and illness, irregular heartbeat, numbness or tingling in hands, feet, or lips, shortness of breath or difficult breathing, severe stomach pain with nausea and vomiting, unexplained nervousness, unusual tiredness or weakness, weakness or heaviness of legs, weight loss.

Immediately notify your Doctor if any of the following side effects appear:

Blood in urine, flushing of face and neck (for injection only), wheezing or shortness of breath (for injection only).

Toxicity and adverse reactions:

Because of the way that Cyclosporine acts on the body, there is a chance that it may cause effects years after the medicine is used. These delayed effects may include certain types of cancer, such as lymphomas or skin cancers. You and your doctor should discuss the good this medicine will do as well as the risks of using it.

Cytotec (Misoprostol)

Check with your Doctor if any of the following side effects appear:

Abdominal cramps, diarrhea, and/or nausea, especially during the first few weeks of treatment. (These side effects may disappear as your body gets used to the drug).

Always notify your Doctor if any of the following side effects appear:

Constipation, gas, indigestion, headache, heavy menstrual bleeding, menstrual disorder, menstrual pain or cramps, paleness, spotting or light bleeding between menstrual periods, stomach or intestinal bleeding, vomiting.

Immediately notify your Doctor if any of the following side effects appear:

Severe diarrhea, severe cramping, or severe nausea.

The following symptoms are symptoms of an overdose. Notify your Doctor immediately:

Extended abdominal pain, breathing difficulty, convulsions, diarrhea lasting more than 2 days, fever, heart palpitations, low blood pressure, sedation or extreme drowsiness, slowed heartbeat, severe stomach or intestinal discomfort, tremors.

Toxicity and adverse reactions:

Cytotec is a synthetic prostaglandin, which is a hormone-like substance. It reduces the production of stomach acid and protects the stomach lining. Do not take Cytotec if you are sensitive to or have ever had an allergic reaction to it or to another prostaglandin medication.

If you are given Cytotec tablets to help prevent stomach ulcers during NSAID treatment, take Cytotec with meals, exactly as prescribed, and for the full course of NSAID treatment, even if you notice no stomach problems. Always take the final dosage at bedtime.

Cytotec may cause uterine bleeding even if you have gone through menopause.

Important Notes for all Women:

Postmenopausal bleeding could be a sign of some other gynecological problem. If you experience any such bleeding while taking Cytotec, notify your doctor at once.

Do not take Cytotec if you are pregnant or might become pregnant while taking it.

If you are pregnant or plan to become pregnant, inform your Doctor immediately. Cytotec can cause dangerous cases of miscarriage that can sometimes lead to the mother's death. Cytotec should not be taken during pregnancy.

If you are a woman of childbearing age, you should not take Cytotec unless you have thoroughly discussed the risks with your Doctor and believe you are able to take effective contraceptive measures.

You will need to take a pregnancy test about 2 weeks before starting to take Cytotec. To be sure you are not pregnant at the start of Cytotec treatment, your Doctor should have you take your first dose on the second or third day of your menstrual period.

Even the most well planned out contraceptive measures sometimes fail. If you believe you may have become pregnant while taking Cytotec, stop taking the drug and contact your Doctor immediately.

Because of the potential for severe diarrhea in a nursing infant, your Doctor may have you stop breastfeeding until your treatment is finished.

Dapsone

Check with your Doctor if any of the following side effects appear:

Gastrointestinal upset including nausea or vomiting, headache, blue discoloration of lips and fingertips.

Always notify your Doctor if any of the following side effects appear:

Anemia, tiredness, shortness of breath, widespread skin rash, weakness of the foot and hand muscles, psychosis, which are hallucinations or delusions.

Immediately notify your Doctor in any of the following side effects appear:

Fever, sore throat, skin infections, or other local signs of infection, severe fatigue, fever, sore throat, rash and prominent lymph glands.

Toxicity and adverse reactions:

Your Doctor will monitor you closely while you are taking this medication so you must follow their instructions carefully, and let them know if you start any new medications. Once per week it is advisable to test your ability to walk on your tip-toes and to test your hand grip strength.

You should not take this medication if you are allergic to it. Let your Doctor know if you are allergic to sulfur antibiotics. Also, if you have significant heart or lung disease, the dose may have to be lower because of the drug's effect on oxygen carrying capacity of your blood cells. Dapsone should be avoided during pregnancy and breast-feeding.

Usually, a blood test is performed as a base line before starting Dapsone. It is then checked after about a week on therapy, and then about once a month, depending on the dose and state of the blood count. It is important that you follow instructions precisely regarding the timing of these tests.

Decadron Tablets (Dexamethasone)

Check with your Doctor if any of the following side effects appear:

Abdominal distention, allergic reactions, bruises, fluid and salt retention, general feeling of illness, glaucoma, headache, hiccups, high blood pressure, hives, increased appetite, peptic ulcer, weight gain.

Always notify your Doctor if any of the following side effects appear:

Increased eye pressure, increased pressure in head, increased sweating, increases in amounts of insulin or hypoglycemic medications needed in diabetes, inflammation of the esophagus, inflammation of the pancreas, irregular menstruation, loss of muscle mass, low potassium levels in blood (leading to symptoms such as dry mouth, excessive thirst, weak or irregular heartbeat, and muscle pain or cramps), muscle weakness, nausea, osteoporosis.

Immediately notify your Doctor if any of the following side effects appear:

Blood clots, bone fractures and degeneration, cataracts, congestive heart failure, convulsions, sings of Cushing's syndrome, high blood pressure, emotional disturbances, excessive hairiness perforated small and large bowel, poor healing of wounds, protruding eyeballs, suppression of growth in children, thin skin, tiny red or purplish spots on the skin, torn tendons, vertigo.

Toxicity and adverse reactions:

Decadron lowers your resistance to infections and can make them harder to treat and may also mask some of the signs of an infection, making it difficult for your doctor to diagnose the actual problem.

If you are taking large doses of this medication, your Doctor may advise you to take it with meals and to take antacids between meals to prevent a peptic ulcer from developing.

Check with your doctor before stopping Decadron abruptly. If you have been taking the medication for a long time, you may need to reduce your dose gradually over a period of days or weeks. The lowest possible dose should always be used, and as symptoms subside, dosage should be reduced gradually.

Decadron should not be used if you have a fungal infection, or if you are sensitive or allergic to any of its ingredients.

Do not get a smallpox vaccination or any other immunizations while taking Decadron, especially in high doses. The vaccination might not take, and could do harm to the nervous system.

If you have an allergy to any cortisone-like drug, Cirrhosis, Diabetes, Diverticulitis, eye infection, Glaucoma, high blood pressure, impaired thyroid function, kidney disease, a muscle disorder known as Myasthenia gravis, Osteoporosis, Peptic ulcer, recent heart attack, Tuberculosis, Crohn's disease or ulcerative colitis; make sure you notify your Doctor before you begin taking this medication.

It is especially important to check with your doctor before combining Decadron with Aspirin, Coumadin, Ephedrine drugs such as Marax and Rynatuss, Indomethacin (Indocin), Phenobarbital, Phenytoin (Dilantin), Rifampin (Rifadin, Rimactane), and HydroDIURIL.

Dicyclomine hydrochloride (Bentyl)

Check with your Doctor if any of the following side effects appear:

Constipation, decreased sweating, dryness of mouth, nose, throat, or skin, bloated feeling, blurred vision, decreased flow of breast milk, difficulty in urination, difficulty in swallowing, drowsiness, increased sensitivity of eyes to light, lightheadedness, headache, loss of memory, nausea, upset stomach or vomiting, redness/irritation injection site, unusual tiredness or weakness.

Always notify your Doctor if any of the following side effects appear:

Confusion, dizziness, continuing lightheadedness, fainting, eye pain, skin rash or hives.

The following symptoms are symptoms of an overdose. Notify your Doctor immediately:

Continued blurred vision or changes in near vision, clumsiness or unsteadiness, difficulty in breathing, severe muscle weakness, tiredness, dizziness, severe drowsiness, dryness of mouth, nose, or severe sore throat, fast heartbeat, fever, hallucinations, confusion, nervousness, restlessness, irritability, seizures, slurred speech, unusual excitement, unusual warmth, dryness, and flushing of skin.

Toxicity and adverse reactions:

You should use this medication with caution if you have autonomic neuropathy, which is a nerve disorder; liver or kidney disease; hyperthyroidism; high blood pressure; coronary heart disease; congestive heart failure; rapid, irregular heartbeat; hiatal hernia, which is a protrusion of part of the stomach through the diaphragm; or enlargement of the prostate gland.

It is especially important to check with your Doctor before combining Bentyl with Proventil and Ventolin, Amantadine (Symmetrel), Maalox, Quinidex, Pilopine, Tavist, Benzodiazepines (tranquilizers) such as Valium and Xanax, Corticosteroids, Digoxin, Lanoxin, Mellaril and Thorazine, Antidepressants, such as Nardil and Parnate), Metoclopramide, Reglan, Narcotic analgesics, Demerol, Nitrates, Nitroglycerin, Elavil and Tofranil

Dilaudid (Hydromorphone hydrochloride)

Check with your Doctor if any of the following side effects appear:

Anxiety, constipation, dizziness, drowsiness, fear, impairment of mental and physical performance, inability to urinate, mental clouding, mood changes, nausea, restlessness, sedation, sluggishness, troubled and slowed breathing, vomiting.

Always notify your Doctor if any of the following side effects appear:

Agitation, chills, cramps, diarrhea, difficulty urinating, dry mouth, flushing, hallucinations, headache, increased pressure in the head, insomnia, involuntary eye movements, itching, loss of appetite, low or high blood pressure, muscle rigidity or tremor, rashes, shock, slow or rapid heartbeat, small pupils, sweating, taste changes, visual disturbances, weakness.

Immediately notify your Doctor if any of the following side effects appear:

Blurred vision, disorientation, double vision, exaggerated feelings of depression or well-being, failure of breathing or heartbeat, faintness/fainting, light-headedness, muscle spasms of the throat or air passages, palpitations, sudden dizziness on standing, tingling and/or numbness, tremor, uncoordinated muscle movements.

The following symptoms are symptoms of an overdose. Notify your Doctor immediately:

Bluish tinge to skin, cold and clammy skin, constricted pupils, coma, extreme sleepiness progressing to a state of unresponsiveness, labored

224

or slowed breathing, limp, weak muscles, low blood pressure, slow heart rate.

With severe overdose, the patient may stop breathing, go into shock, or have a heart attack; and death can occur.

Toxicity and adverse reactions:

This medication is habit forming.

If you are sensitive to or have ever had an allergic reaction to narcotic painkillers you should not take this medication.

Dilaudid should be used with caution if you are in a weakened condition or if you have a severe liver or kidney disorder, hypothyroidism, Addison's disease, commonly referred to as adrenal gland failure, an enlarged prostate, a urethral stricture, low blood pressure or a head injury.

Dilaudid suppresses the cough reflex. Your Doctor will be cautious about prescribing this medication after an operation or for patients with a lung disease.

Narcotics such as Dilaudid may mask or hide the symptoms of sudden or severe abdominal conditions, making diagnosis and treatment difficult.

Dilaudid can cause seizures when taken in high doses and, if you have a seizure disorder, can make the seizures worse.

Do not drink alcohol while taking this medication.

It is especially important to check with your doctor before combining Dilaudid with Antiemetics such as Compazine and Phenergan, Antihistamines, general anesthetics, Nembutal, Restoril, Demerol and Percocet, Phenothiazines such as Thorazine, Sedative/hypnotics such as Valium, Halcion, Tranquilizers such as Xanax, Tricyclic antidepressants such as Elavil and Tofranil

Dipentum (Olsalazine sodium)

Check with your Doctor if any of the following side effects appear:

Abdominal or stomach pain or upset, diarrhea, loss of appetite, aching joints and muscles, acne, anxiety or depression, dizziness or drowsiness, headache, trouble in sleeping.

Immediately notify your Doctor if any of the following side effects appear:

Back or stomach pain (severe), bloody diarrhea, fast heartbeat, fever, nausea or vomiting, skin rash, swelling of the stomach, yellow eyes or skin.

Toxicity and adverse reactions:

If you have kidney disease, Dipentum could cause further damage. You will need regular checks on your kidney function, so be sure to keep all regular appointments with your Doctor.

You should not be using Dipentum if you are allergic to salicylates such as aspirin.

It is especially important to check with your doctor before combining Dipentum with Coumadin.

Donnatal (Phenobarbital, Hyoscyamine sulfate, Atropine sulfate, Scopolamine hydrobromide, Bellatal)

Check with your Doctor if any of the following side effects appear:

Constipation, decreased sweating, dizziness, drowsiness, dryness of mouth, nose, throat, or skin, bloated feeling, blurred vision, decreased flow of breast milk, difficult urination, difficulty in swallowing, headache, increased sensitivity of eyes to sunlight, loss of memory, nausea or vomiting, unusual tiredness or weakness.

Always notify your Doctor if any of the following side effects appear:

Eye pain, skin rash or hives, sore throat and fever, unusual bleeding or bruising, yellow eyes or skin, diarrhea, especially if you have an ileostomy or colostomy.

The following symptoms are symptoms of an overdose. Notify your Doctor immediately:

Continuing blurred vision or changes in near vision, clumsiness, unsteadiness, confusion, convulsions, seizures, continuing dizziness, severe drowsiness, dryness of mouth, nose, or severe sore throat, fast heartbeat, fever, hallucinations, shortness of breath or troubled breathing, slurred speech, unusual excitement, nervousness, restlessness, or irritability, unusual warmth, dryness, and flushing of skin.

Toxicity and adverse reactions:

Donnatal may intensify the effects of alcohol. Avoid taking antacids within 1 hour of a dose of Donnatal as they may reduce this medication's effectiveness.

Be cautious in using Donnatal if you suffer from high blood pressure, hyperthyroidism, irregular or rapid heartbeat, or heart, kidney, or liver disease. Donnatal can decrease sweating so if you are exercising or are subjected to high temperatures, be alert for heat exhaustion or heat stroke.

If you have a gastric ulcer, use this medication with caution.

It is especially important to check with your doctor before combining Donnatal with Antidepressants, Antihistamines, Bentyl, Cogentin, Barbiturates, Coumadin, Diarrhea medications containing Kaolin or Attapulgite, Digitalis (Lanoxin), Narcotic medications, Potassium, Corticosteroids, and Tranquilizers.

Elocon (Mometasone furoate)

Check with your Doctor if any of the following side effects appear:

Acne-like pimples, allergic skin rash, boils, burning, damaged skin, dryness, excessive hairiness, infected hair follicles, infection of the skin, irritation, itching, light colored patches on skin, prickly heat, rash around the mouth, skin atrophy and wasting, softening of the skin, stretch marks, tingling or stinging.

Toxicity and adverse reactions:

Elocon is for use only on the skin. Be careful to keep it out of your eyes.

Be careful not to use Elocon for a longer time than prescribed. If you do, you may disrupt your ability to make your own natural adrenal corticoid hormones. If your condition doesn't improve in 2 weeks, call your Doctor.

Do not use Elocon if you have ever had an allergic reaction to it or any other steroid medication.

If you have any kind of skin infection, tell your Doctor before you start using Elocon.

Do not use Elocon cream or ointment on your face, underarms, or groin area unless your Doctor gives you specific instructions to do so.

Extensive or long-term use of Elocon may cause Cushing's syndrome.

Enbrel (Etanercept)

Always notify your Doctor if any of the following side effects appear:

Abdominal pain, cough, dizziness, headache, indigestion, infections, injection site reaction, nausea, rash, respiratory problems, respiratory tract infection, sinus and nasal inflammation, sore throat, vomiting, weakness.

Immediately notify your Doctor if any of the following side effects appear:

Abscess, altered sense of taste, blood clots, blood disorders and infections, bursitis, chest pain, depression, diarrhea, difficulty breathing, dry eyes, dry mouth, fatigue, fever, flu-like symptoms, flushing, gallbladder problems, hair loss, heart attack, heart failure, high or low blood pressure, hives, inflammation in the digestive tract, intestinal perforation, itching, joint pain, kidney inflammation, loss of appetite, mouth sores, pain, nerve damage, raised patches of red skin (lupus), red eyes, seizures, stomach and intestinal bleeding, stroke, swelling in the arms or legs, swollen face and throat, tingling or burning sensation, urinary tract infection, vision loss, weight gain.

Toxicity and adverse reactions:

Enbrel can be taken along with other medications commonly used to treat rheumatoid arthritis, including Methotrexate (Rheumatrex), Corticosteroids, NSAID's, and other pain-killers.

Tumor Necrosis Factor plays a significant role in the immune system, so blocking its action can lower your resistance to infection. Serious, and even fatal infections have been known to occur, especially in people whose immune systems have already been weakened by advancing age, conditions such as heart failure or diabetes, or medications such as Imuran, Prograf, Cellcept, Neoral, and Sandimmune.

For the same reason, children with juvenile rheumatoid arthritis should be brought up to date with all immunizations before starting Enbrel therapy.

Enbrel is given by injection under the skin of the thigh, abdomen, or upper arm. Your Doctor will instruct you in the proper drug preparation and injection technique and supervise your first injection in the office. You should rotate injection sites and make each new injection at least 1 inch from an older one. Never inject into areas where the skin is tender, bruised, red, or hard.

Do not shake Enbrel solution. Avoid handling the needle cover if you have a latex allergy. *Never reuse a syringe.*

If Enbrel gives you an allergic reaction, you will not be able to continue using it. Do not start taking it during any kind of infection.

Think carefully about using this medication if you are prone to repeated infections or have a condition that encourages infections, such as diabetes or Crohn's disease. Be cautious, too, if you have a disease of the nervous system such as multiple sclerosis or a seizure disorder; such problems have been known to develop or get worse during Enbrel therapy. Enbrel should also be used with caution if you are prone to blood disorders, since they have occasionally appeared during treatment with Enbrel.

If you develop an infection, stop taking Enbrel and call your doctor immediately. Do likewise if you are exposed to chickenpox.

Do not get any live-type vaccinations while taking Enbrel.

Dosage is determined by weight. The safety of Enbrel has not been studied in children less than 4 years old.

Entocort

Check with your Doctor if any of the following side effects appear:

Fluid retention, weight gain, headache, muscle weakness.

Notify your Doctor in any of the following side effects appear:

Stomach pain, nausea or vomiting.

Immediately notify your Doctor if any of the following side effects appear:

Irregular menses, convulsions, seizures, blurred vision, sever stomach pain.

Erythromycin, Oral (E.E.S., E-Mycin, ERYC, Ery-Tab, Erythrocin, PCE)

Check with your Doctor if any of the following side effects appear:

Abdominal pain, diarrhea, loss of appetite, nausea, vomiting.

Always notify your Doctor if any of the following side effects appear:

Hives, rash, skin eruptions, jaundice.

Immediately notify your Doctor if any of the following side effects appear:

Hearing loss (temporary), inflammation of the large intestine, irregular heartbeat, severe allergic reaction, severe blisters in the mouth and eyes, skin reddening.

The following symptoms are symptoms of an overdose. Notify your Doctor immediately:

Diarrhea, nausea, stomach cramps, vomiting.

Toxicity and adverse reactions:

If you have ever had liver disease, consult your Doctor before taking Erythromycin. This medication may cause severe intestinal inflammation.

If a new infection develops, called a superinfection, immediately notify your Doctor because you may need to be treated with a different antibiotic. Prolonged or repeated use of Erythromycin may result in the growth of bacteria or fungi that do not respond to this medication and can cause a second infection.

Combining erythromycin with Lovastatin (Mevacor) can cause severe muscle wasting and damage to the kidneys. If you are taking both of these medications, your Doctor will monitor you closely for warning signs of this interaction. If you have muscle weakness known as Myasthenia gravis, it can be aggravated by Erythromycin.

It is especially important to check with your doctor before combining Erythromycin with Benzodiazepines such as Halcion and Versed, Coumadin, Bromocriptine (Parlodel), Carbamazepine (Tegretol), Cyclosporine (Sandimmune, Neoral), Digoxin (Lanoxin), Dihydroergotamine (D.H.E. 45), Disopyramide (Norpace), Ergotamine (Cafergot), Hexobarbital Seizure medications such as Depakene, Depakote, and Dilantin, Tacrolimus (Prograf), Theophylline (Theo-Dur).

Flagyl (Metronidazole)

Check with your Doctor if any of the following side effects appear:

Diarrhea, dizziness or lightheadedness, headache, loss of appetite, stomach pain or cramps, change in taste sensation, dryness of mouth, unpleasant or sharp metallic taste, any vaginal irritation, discharge, or dryness not present before use of this medicine, mood or other mental changes, skin rash, hives, redness, or itching, sore throat and fever, severe stomach or back pain.

For injection form, check with your Doctor if the following side effect appears:

Pain, tenderness, redness, or swelling over vein in which the medicine is given.

234

Immediately notify your Doctor if any of the following side effects appear:

Numbness, tingling, pain, or weakness in hands or feet, convulsions, seizures.

The following symptoms are symptoms of an overdose. Notify your Doctor immediately.

Lack of muscle coordination, nausea, vomiting.

Toxicity and adverse reactions:

Flagyl may cause dark urine in some patients. This is temporary and will go away when you stop taking this medicine.

It is especially important to check with your doctor before combining Flagyl with Coumadin, Cholestyramine (Questran), Cimetidine (Tagamet), Disulfiram (Antabuse), Lithium, Phenobarbital, Phenytoin (Dilantin).

Do not take Flagyl if you have ever had an allergic reaction to or are sensitive to Metronidazole or similar drugs.

Fosamax (Alendronate sodium)

Check with your Doctor if any of the following side effects appear:

Abdominal pain, bone and joint pain, constipation, diarrhea, indigestion, muscle pain, nausea.

Always notify your Doctor if any of the following side effects appear:

Abdominal distention, acid backup, difficulty in swallowing, esophageal ulcers, gas, headache, stomach ulcers, vomiting.

Immediately notify your Doctor if any of the following side effects appear:

Changes in taste, esophageal blockage or perforation, eye pain, hives, inflammation of the stomach, mouth sores, muscle cramps, rash, skin redness, swollen face and throat.

The following symptoms are symptoms of an overdose. Notify your Doctor immediately:

Heartburn, inflammation of the esophagus or stomach, ulcer, upset stomach.

Toxicity and adverse reactions:

Fosamax is effective only when each tablet is taken with a full glass of plain water first thing in the morning, at least 30 minutes before the first food, beverage, or other medication. If you can wait longer before eating or drinking, the medication will be absorbed better. Do not lie down for at least 30 minutes after taking Fosamax and avoid chewing or sucking on the tablet because it can cause mouth sores.

You should take calcium and vitamin D supplements if you don't get enough in your diet and avoid smoking as well as alcohol. Fosamax is not recommended for women on hormone replacement therapy, or for women with kidney problems.

Combining aspirin with a Fosamax dose of more than 10 milligrams per day will increase the likelihood of stomach upset. Calcium supplements such as Caltrate, antacids such as Riopan, and some other oral medications will interfere with the absorption of Fosamax, so wait at least 30 minutes after taking Fosamax before you take anything else.

The medication is not recommended for nursing mothers.

Helidac Therapy (Bismuth subsalicylate, Metronidazole, Tetracycline hydrochloride)

Check with your Doctor if any of the following side effects appear:

Abdominal pain, diarrhea, nausea,   ringing in the ears.

Always notify your Doctor if any of the following side effects appear:

Abnormal stools, abnormal taste, appetite loss, black bowel movements, bleeding in stomach or intestines, constipation, discolored tongue, dizziness, duodenal ulcers, gas, headache, indigestion, insomnia, pain, prickly feeling, rectal discomfort, sinus inflammation, upper respiratory infection, vomiting, weakness.

Immediately notify your Doctor if any of the following side effects appear:

Abnormal growths, acne, arthritis, belching, chest pain, conjunctivitis (pinkeye), drowsiness, dry mouth, fainting, flu-like symptoms, general feeling of illness, heart attack, high blood pressure, infection in stomach or intestines, infections, inflamed mouth or tongue, intestinal obstruction, itching, nasal inflammation, nervousness, rash, rectal bleeding, sensitivity to light, skin hemorrhage, stroke, tendon inflammation, tooth problems, trouble swallowing, urinary tract infection.

The following symptoms are symptoms of an overdose. Notify your Doctor immediately:

An overdose of the Bismuth subsalicylate part of Helidac Therapy can be fatal.

Confusion, coma, convulsions, coordination problems, diarrhea, fast heartbeat, high fever, lethargy, nausea, numbness or pain in the arms and legs, rapid breathing, ringing in the ears, severe heart and lung problems, vomiting.

Toxicity and adverse reactions:

There are four pills in each dose of Helidac Therapy. The two pink tablets (Bismuth subsalicylate) should be chewed and swallowed. The white tablet (Metronidazole) and the orange and white capsule (Tetracycline) should be swallowed whole. Be sure to drink at least 8 ounces of fluid with each dose, especially at bedtime, to prevent irritation.

You should also be taking an acid blocker such as Zantac, Pepcid, or Tagamet.

238

Do not take Helidac Therapy if you have ever had an allergic reaction to Aspirin, Pepto-Bismol, Flagyl, Tetracycline or Vibramycin.

Helidac Therapy is not for use by children and pregnant or nursing women. The Tetracycline part of the therapy can harm a developing baby, stunt a child's growth, and interfere with tooth development.

You should avoid Helidac Therapy if you have kidney or liver disease.

Don't be alarmed if your tongue and/or bowel movements turn black while you are taking Helidac Therapy. This is a harmless side effect of the Bismuth subsalicylate part of the therapy.

Combining aspirin with Helidac Therapy sometimes causes ringing in the ears. If this happens, check with your Doctor. You may need to temporarily stop taking aspirin.

During Helidac Therapy, alcoholic beverages can cause abdominal cramps, nausea, vomiting, headache, and flushing. Avoid alcohol until at least 1 day after finishing Helidac.

For 1 hour before and 2 hours after each dose of Helidac Therapy, avoid eating dairy products as they can interfere with the medication's absorption.

Since Helidac Therapy can interfere with oral contraceptives, you should use an additional form of birth control during Helidac Therapy.

Do not start Helidac Therapy if you have taken the anti-alcohol drug Antabuse within the past 2 weeks. Certain other drugs may also adversely interact with this medication. Check with your doctor before combining Helidac Therapy with Antacids containing aluminum, calcium, or magnesium, Coumadin, Tagamet, Diabetes medications such as insulin and glyburide (Micronase), Iron (including vitamins that contain iron), Lithium (Eskalith, Lithobid), Penicillin, Phenobarbital, Phenytoin (Dilantin), Probenecid (Benemid), Sodium bicarbonate (baking soda), Sulfinpyrazone (Anturane), and Zinc (including vitamins that contain zinc).

Do not undertake Helidac Therapy if you are pregnant or breastfeeding.

Hydrocortisone Skin Preparations (Cetacort, Hytone, Nutracort)

Check with your Doctor if any of the following side effects appear:

Acne-like skin eruptions, burning, dryness, growth of excessive hair, inflammation of the hair follicles, inflammation around the mouth, irritation, itching, peeling skin, prickly heat, secondary infection, skin inflammation, skin softening, stretch marks, unusual lack of skin color.

The following symptoms are symptoms of an overdose. Notify your Doctor immediately:

Glandular problems, higher than normal amounts of sugar in the blood, and high amounts of sugar in the urine.

Toxicity and adverse reactions:

When you apply a hydrocortisone cream or lotion, you will inevitably absorb some of the medication through your skin and into the bloodstream. Too much absorption can lead to unwanted side effects elsewhere in the body so to keep this problem to a minimum, avoid using large amounts of hydrocortisone over extensive areas, and do not cover it with airtight dressings such as plastic wrap or adhesive bandages unless specifically told to by your Doctor.

Hydrocortisone cream and lotion are for use only on the skin. Be careful to keep them out of your eyes.

If you are using hydrocortisone for psoriasis or a condition that has been difficult to cure, your Doctor may advise you to use a bandage or covering over the affected area. If an infection develops, remove the bandage and contact your Doctor.

If you use this medication over large areas of skin for prolonged periods of time or cover the treated area, the amount of the hormone absorbed into your bloodstream may eventually lead to Cushing's syndrome. You can also develop glandular problems or high blood sugar, or show sugar in your urine.

Children, because of their relatively larger ratio of skin surface area to body weight, are particularly susceptible to over absorption of hydrocortisone.

241

Long-term treatment of children with steroids such as hydrocortisone may interfere with growth and development.

Imodium (Loperamide hydrochloride)

Check with your Doctor if any of the following side effects appear:

Abdominal distention, abdominal pain or discomfort, allergic reactions, including skin rash, constipation, dizziness, drowsiness, dry mouth, nausea and vomiting, tiredness.

Immediately notify your Doctor if any of the following side effects appear:

Continuing diarrhea (2 days or more), bloody stools, fever.

The following symptoms are symptoms of an overdose. Notify your Doctor immediately:

Constipation, drowsiness, lethargy and depression, nausea.

Toxicity and adverse reactions:

While using Imodium, you should exercise extra caution while driving or performing tasks requiring mental alertness.

Imodium is not good for all types of diarrhea. It is not prescribed for acute dysentery, which is an inflammation of the intestines characterized by abdominal pain; watery/sometimes bloody stools; and fever, caused by bacteria, viruses, or parasites.

Dehydration can be a problem when you have diarrhea so it is important that you drink plenty of fluids while taking Imodium.

Use special caution when giving Imodium to a young child because their response to the medication can be unpredictable.

If you have a liver problem, your Doctor should closely watch for signs of central nervous system reactions, such as drowsiness or convulsions.

Infliximab (Remicade)

Always notify your Doctor if any of the following side effects appear:

Abdominal pain, cough, dizziness, fainting, headache, muscle pain, nasal congestion, nausea, runny nose, shortness of breath, sneezing, sore throat, tightness in chest, unusual tiredness or weakness, vomiting, wheezing, back pain, bloody or cloudy urine, cracks in skin at the corners of mouth, diarrhea difficult or painful urination, frequent urge to urinate, high blood pressure, low blood pressure, pain, pain or tenderness around eyes and cheekbones, skin, rash, soreness or irritation of mouth or tongue, soreness or redness around fingernails or toenails, vaginal burning or itching and discharge, white patches in mouth and/or on tongue, abscess, back or side pain, black, tarry stools, blood in urine or stools, bone or joint pain, constipation, falls, feeling of fullness.

243

Always notify your Doctor if any of the following side effects appear:

Hernia (bulge of tissue through the wall of the abdomen), infection, irregular or pounding heartbeat, pain in rectum, pain spreading from the abdomen to the left shoulder, pinpoint red spots on skin, severe stomach pain, swollen or painful glands, tendon injury, unusual bleeding or bruising, unusual weight loss, yellow skin and eyes

Immediately notify your Doctor if any of the following side effects appear:

Chest pain, chills, fever, flushing of face, hives, itching, troubled breathing

Levsin (Hycoscyamine sulfate, Anaspaz, Levbid, Levsinex)

Check with your Doctor if any of the following side effects appear:

Constipation (less common with hyoscyamine), decreased sweating, dryness of mouth, nose, throat, or skin, bloated feeling, blurred vision, decreased flow of breast milk, difficult urination, difficulty in swallowing, drowsiness, headache, increased sensitivity of eyes to light, lightheadedness (with injection), loss of memory, nausea or vomiting, redness or other signs of irritation at place of injection, unusual tiredness or weakness.

Always notify your Doctor if any of the following side effects appear:

244

Confusion (especially in the elderly), dizziness, continuing lightheadedness, fainting, eye pain, skin rash or hives.

The following symptoms are symptoms of an overdose. Notify your Doctor immediately:

Continuing blurred vision or changes in near vision, clumsiness or unsteadiness, confusion, convulsions, seizures, difficulty in breathing, severe muscle weakness, severe tiredness, dizziness, severe drowsiness, dryness of mouth, nose, or severe sore throat, fast heartbeat, fever, hallucinations, slurred speech, unusual excitement, nervousness, restlessness, or irritability, unusual warmth, dryness, and flushing of skin.

Toxicity and adverse reactions:

Levsin may make you sweat less, causing your body temperature to increase and putting you at the risk of heatstroke. Try to stay inside as much as possible on hot days, and avoid warm places such as very hot baths and saunas.

You should not be given Levsin if you have bowel or digestive tract obstruction or paralysis, glaucoma; a muscle disorder called Myasthenia gravis, ulcerative colitis or urinary obstruction.

Levsin is not appropriate if you have diarrhea, especially if you have an ileostomy or colostomy and be careful using Levsin if you have an overactive thyroid gland, heart disease, congestive heart failure, irregular heartbeats, high blood pressure, or kidney disease.

While you are taking Levsin, you may experience confusion, disorientation, short-term memory loss, hallucinations, difficulty speaking, lack of coordination, coma, an exaggerated sense of well-being, decreased anxiety, fatigue, sleeplessness and agitation. These symptoms should disappear 12 to 48 hours after you stop taking the drug. Because Levsin may make you dizzy or drowsy, or blur your vision, do not drive, operate other machinery, or do any other hazardous work while taking this medication.

It is especially important to check with your doctor before combining Levsin with Amantadine (Symmetrel), Antacids, Elavil, Nardil, Parnate, Tofranil, Benadryl, Thorazine, Haldol, Bentyl or Potassium supplements such as Slow-K.

Librax

Check with your Doctor if any of the following side effects appear:

Bloated feeling, nausea, decreased sweating, dizziness, drowsiness, dryness of mouth, headache, blurred vision, decreased sexual ability, loss of memory, unusual tiredness or weakness.

Always notify your Doctor if any of the following side effects appear:

Constipation, eye pain, mental depression, skin rash or hives, slow heartbeat, shortness of breath, or troubled breathing, sore throat and fever, trouble in sleeping, unusual excitement, nervousness, or irritability, yellow eyes or skin.

The following symptoms are symptoms of an overdose. Notify your Doctor immediately:

Confusion, difficult urination, severe drowsiness, dryness of mouth, nose, or severe sore throat, fast heartbeat, unusual warmth, dryness, and flushing of skin.

After you stop using this medicine, check with your Doctor if any of the following side effects appear:

Convulsions, seizures, muscle cramps, nausea or vomiting, stomach cramps, trembling.

Toxicity and adverse reactions:

<u>Librax can be habit-forming.</u>

You should not take Librax drug if you have glaucoma, an enlarged prostate called Prostatic hypertrophy, or a bladder obstruction.

You should not stop taking Librax suddenly, because of the risk of withdrawal symptoms such as convulsions, cramps, tremors, vomiting, sweating, feeling depressed, and insomnia. If you have been taking Librax over a long period of time, your Doctor will have you taper off gradually.

The elderly are more likely to develop side effects such as confusion, excessive drowsiness, and uncoordinated movements when taking Librax. Your Doctor will probably prescribe a low dose.

Long-term treatment with Librax may call for periodic blood and liver function tests.

It is especially important to check with your Doctor before combining Librax with MAO inhibitors such as Nardil and Parnate, Coumadin, Donnagel, Kaopectate, Ketoconazole (Nizoral), Stelazine and Thorazine, or Potassium supplements such as Micro-K. You may experience excessive drowsiness and other potentially dangerous side effects if you combine Librax with alcohol or other drugs, such as Benadryl and Valium.

Librax is rarely recommended for use by pregnant women because several studies have found an increased risk of birth defects if it is taken during the first 3 months of pregnancy. Due to the severe risk to your unborn fetus, if you are pregnant, plan to become pregnant, or are breastfeeding, inform your Doctor immediately.

Lidex (Fluocinonide)

Check with your Doctor if any of the following side effects appear:

Acne-like eruptions, burning, dryness, excessive hair growth, infection of the skin, irritation, itching, lack of skin color, prickly heat, skin inflammation, skin loss or softening, stretch marks.

Toxicity and adverse reactions:

Lidex is for use only on the skin so be very careful to keep it out of your eyes. If the medication gets in your eyes and causes irritation, immediately flush your eyes with a large amount of water.

You should not be using Lidex if you are allergic to any of its components.

If enough of the drug is absorbed through the skin, it may produce unusual side effects, including increased sugar in your blood and urine and Cushing's syndrome.

Children may absorb a proportionally greater amount of steroid drugs and may be more sensitive to the effects of these drugs. Effects experienced by children may include bulges on the head, delayed weight gain, headache and slow growth.

Extended treatment time with any steroid product may cause skin to waste away. This may also occur with short-term use on the face, armpits, and skin creases.

Lidex can be absorbed in amounts large enough to have temporary effects on the adrenal, hypothalamic, and pituitary glands

Lomotil (Diphenoxylate hydrochloride, Atropine sulfate)

Check with your Doctor if any of the following side effects appear:

Blurred vision, confusion, difficult urination, dizziness or lightheadedness, drowsiness, dryness of skin and mouth, fever, headache, mental depression, numbness of hands or feet, skin rash or itching, swelling of the gums.

Always notify your Doctor if any of the following side effects appear. The following side effects may be sever and occur suddenly. If this happens, call your Doctor immediately, since this may be signs of a more severe and dangerous problem with your bowels.

Bloating, constipation, loss of appetite, severe stomach pain with nausea and vomiting

The following symptoms are symptoms of an overdose. Notify your Doctor immediately:

Continuing blurred vision or changes in near vision, severe drowsiness, dryness of mouth, nose, and severe sore throat, fast heartbeat, shortness of breath or severe troubled breathing, unusual excitement, nervousness, restlessness, or irritability, unusual warmth, dryness, and flushing of the skin.

Toxicity and adverse reactions:

Lomotil is not recommended in children under 2 years of age.

It is especially important to check with your doctor before combining Lomotil with Barbiturates, Anticonvulsants and sedatives such as Phenobarbital, Antidepressants such as Nardil and Parnate, and Tranquilizers such as Valium and Xanax. Lomotil may intensify the effects of alcohol.

250

Unless you are directed to do so by your doctor, do not take Lomotil if you have obstructive jaundice, which is a disease in which bile made in the liver does not reach the intestines because of a bile duct obstruction such as gallstones. Do not take Lomotil if you have diarrhea associated with pseudomembranous enterocolitis, which is an inflammation of the intestines, or an infection with enterotoxin-producing bacteria, which is a poisonous substance that affects the stomach and intestines.

Certain antibiotics such as Ceclor, Cleocin, PCE and Achromycin V may cause diarrhea. Lomotil can make this type of diarrhea worse and longer-lasting. Check with your Doctor before using Lomotil while taking an antibiotic.

Lomotil slows activity of the digestive system, which can result in a buildup of fluid in the intestine. This may worsen the dehydration and imbalance in normal body salts that
usually occur with diarrhea. If you have severe ulcerative colitis, your Doctor will want to monitor your condition while you are taking this drug.

Use Lomotil with extreme caution if you have kidney and liver disease or if your liver is not functioning normally.

Lomotil should be used with caution in children, since side effects may occur even with recommended doses, especially in children with Down's syndrome.

Since addiction to Diphenoxylate hydrochloride is possible at high doses, you should never exceed the recommended dosage.

Lopid (Gemfibrozil)

Check with your Doctor if any of the following side effects appear:

Abdominal pain, acute appendicitis, constipation, diarrhea, eczema, fatigue, headache, indigestion, nausea/vomiting, rash, vertigo.

Always notify your Doctor if any of the following side effects appear:

Anemia, blood disorders, decreased male fertility, decreased sex drive, hives, impotence, itching, joint pain, muscle disease, muscle pain, muscle weakness, painful extremities, sleepiness, tingling sensation, weight loss, jaundice.

Immediately notify your Doctor if any of the following side effects appear:

Burred vision, confusion, convulsions, depression, dizziness, fainting, inflammation of the colon, irregular heartbeat, laryngeal swelling.

The following symptoms are symptoms of an overdose. Notify your Doctor immediately:

Abdominal cramps, diarrhea, joint and muscle pain, nausea, vomiting.

Toxicity and adverse reactions:

Lopid is prescribed, along with a special diet, for treatment of patients with very high levels of serum triglycerides who are at risk of developing pancreatitis, and who do not respond adequately to a strict diet and exercise. This medication can also be used to reduce the risk of coronary heart disease.

It's important to remember that Lopid is a supplement and not a substitute for these other measures. To get the full benefit of the medication, you need to stick to the diet and exercise program prescribed by your Doctor. All of these efforts to keep your cholesterol levels normal are important because together they may lower your risk of heart disease.

There is a slight possibility that Lopid may cause malignancy, gallbladder disease, abdominal pain leading to appendectomy, or other serious, possibly fatal, abdominal disorders. This drug should not be used by those who have only mildly elevated cholesterol levels, since the benefits do not outweigh the risk of these severe side effects.

If you are sensitive to or have ever had an allergic reaction to Lopid or similar drugs such as Atromid-S, you should not take this medication. Make sure your Doctor is aware of any drug reactions you have experienced.

Do not combine Lopid with any of the cholesterol-lowering medications known as "statins," including Lescol, Lipitor, Mevacor, Pravachol, and Zocor. This combination increases the danger of serious, muscle-wasting side effects.

253

Excess body weight and excess alcohol intake may be important risk factors leading to unusually high levels of fats in the body. If you are overweight, your Doctor will probably want you to lose weight and stop drinking before they try to treat you with Lopid.

Your Doctor will probably do periodic blood level tests during the first 12 months of therapy with Lopid because of blood diseases associated with the use of this medication.

If you are being treated for any gallbladder condition or a disease that contributes to increased blood cholesterol, such as an overactive thyroid, diabetes, nephrotic syndrome, which is a kidney and blood vessel disorder, dysproteinemia, which is an excess of protein in the blood, or obstructive liver disease, consult with your Doctor before taking Lopid.

It is important that your Doctor check your progress regularly because Lopid should begin to reduce your cholesterol levels during the first 3 months of therapy. If your cholesterol is not lowered sufficiently, this medication should be discontinued.

Be sure to check with your Doctor before taking Lopid along with Coumadin because the dosage of Coumadin must be reduced to avoid abnormal bleeding.

This drug should be used with caution by older adults.

Medrol (Methylprednisolone)

Check with your Doctor if any of the following side effects appear:

Abdominal swelling, allergic reactions, bone fractures, bruising, cataracts, face redness, fluid and salt retention, headache, increased sweating, mood swings, thin, fragile skin, tiny red or purplish spots on the skin, vertigo.

Always notify your Doctor if any of the following side effects appear:

High blood pressure, glaucoma, muscle wasting and weakness, Osteoporosis, poor healing of wounds.

Immediately notify your Doctor if any of the following side effects appear:

Congestive heart failure, convulsions, Cushing's syndrome, increase in amounts of insulin or hypoglycemic medications needed, inflammation of the pancreas, irregular menstruation, protruding eyes, signs of Tuberculosis, stomach ulcer, suppression of growth in children, symptoms of diabetes.

Toxicity and adverse reactions:

Medrol lowers your resistance to infections and can make them harder to treat and it may also mask some of the signs of an infection, making it difficult for your Doctor to diagnose the source of the infection.

The 24 mg tablet contains FD&C Yellow No. 5 (tartrazine), which has caused allergic reactions, including asthma, in some people. Although this is rare, it is more common in people who are sensitive to aspirin.

You should avoid immunization shots with live or live, attenuated vaccines while taking high doses of Medrol, because Medrol can suppress the immune system. Immunization with killed or inactivated vaccines is safe, but may have diminished effect.

This medication may aggravate existing emotional problems or cause new ones. You may experience euphoria, which is an exaggerated sense of well-being, difficulty in sleeping, mood swings, or mental problems.

Medrol should be taken with caution if you have a fungal infection, Diverticulitis, Crohn's disease, ulcerative colitis, high blood pressure, kidney diseases, Peptic ulcer, a muscle disorder called Myasthenia gravis, Osteoporosis, threadworm, underactive thyroid, Cirrhosis, or herpes simplex infection of the eye.

Medrol can slow the growth and development of infants and children care should be taken to avoid exposure to chickenpox and measles.

It is especially important to check with your Doctor before combining Medrol with Aspirin, Phenobarbital, Coumadin, Carbamazepine (Tegretol), Cyclosporine (Sandimmune, Neoral), Estrogen medications such as Premarin, Insulin, Ketoconazole (Nizoral), NSAID'a, Glucotrol, Phenytoin (Dilantin), Rifampin (Rifadin), Troleandomycin (Tao), Lasix or HydroDIURIL.

Methotrexate (Rheumatrex)

Check with your Doctor if any of the following side effects appear:

Acne, boils, lack of appetite, nausea or vomiting, pale skin, sensitivity to sunlight, itching or rash, temporary hair loss.

Always notify your Doctor if any of the following side effects appear:

Back pain, dark urine, dizziness, drowsiness, headache, unusual weakness or fatigue, yellow eyes or skin (jaundice).

Immediately notify your Doctor if any of the following side effects appear:

Diarrhea, reddening of skin, pinpoint red spots on skin, sores on mouth and lips, stomach pain, allergic reaction, blurred vision, chest pains, confusion, fever or chills, painful peeling of skin patches, dead or loose skin layers, painful or difficult urination, red blisters or ulcers on the lip, mouth, eye, nasal passages, and genital area, reddening of the skin with or without hair loss, seizures, convulsions, shortness of breath, cough, hoarseness or wheezing, side or lower back pain, sloughing of skin, muscle and bone, unusual bleeding or bruising.

Toxicity and adverse reactions:

Be certain to remember that in the treatment of psoriasis and rheumatoid arthritis, Methotrexate is taken once a week, not once a day. Accidentally taking the recommended weekly dosage on a daily basis can lead to fatal overdose.

Methotrexate treatment is not suitable for you if you suffer from psoriasis or rheumatoid arthritis *and* also have abnormal blood cell count, alcoholic liver disease or other chronic liver disease, alcoholism, anemia, HIV or AIDS and you should avoid alcoholic beverages while taking this drug.

Before you start taking this medication, your Doctor should do a chest X-ray plus blood tests to determine your blood cell counts, liver enzyme levels, and the efficiency of your kidney function. While you are taking this medication, the blood tests will be repeated at regular intervals; if you develop a cough or chest pain, the chest X-ray will be repeated.

While you are taking it, you may develop an opportunistic infection, which is an infection that takes advantage of your altered body chemistry. Before receiving any immunization or vaccination, be sure to inform all health care workers that you are taking this drug.

Older or physically debilitated people are particularly vulnerable to toxic effects from this medication. Your Doctor will prescribe the medication with great caution if you have an active infection, liver disease, peptic ulcer or ulcerative colitis.

If you are being given it for the treatment of cancer or psoriasis, you should not take aspirin or other NSAID's as this combination could increase the toxic effects. If you are taking it for rheumatoid arthritis, you may be able to continue taking aspirin or a NSAID, but your Doctor should monitor you carefully. Other drugs that may increase the toxic effects of this medication include Cisplatin (Platinol), Etretinate (Tegison), Penicillin, Phenylbutazone, Phenytoin (Dilantin), Probenecid (Benemid), Bactrim or Gantrisin.

Sulfa drugs may increase the toxic effect on the bone marrow, where new blood cells are made, while certain antibiotics and vitamins containing folic acid may reduce the effectiveness of it. This medication may also alter the effect of Theophylline (Marax, Quibron).

A woman should not start this medication until her Doctor is sure she is not pregnant. Because it causes birth defects and miscarriages, it must not be taken during pregnancy by women with psoriasis or rheumatoid arthritis. It should be taken by women being treated for cancer only if the potential benefit outweighs the risk to the developing baby. Further, a couple should avoid pregnancy if the man taking Methotrexate. After the end of treatment, a man should wait at least 3 months, and a woman should wait for the completion of at least one menstrual cycle, before attempting to conceive a child. Do not take this medication if you are breastfeeding as it does pass into breast milk and may harm a nursing baby.

Nexium (Esomeprazole magnesium)

Check with your Doctor if any of the following side effects appear:

Abdominal pain, diarrhea, headache, burping, change in bowel habits.

Always notify your Doctor if any of the following side effects appear:

Abnormal sense of smell, acne, anemia, apathy, back pain, black stools, chills, dry mouth, loss of appetite, loss of taste.

Immediately notify your Doctor if any of the following side effects appear:

Blood disorders, blood in urine, chest pain, constipation, coughing, cramps, difficulty breathing, difficulty swallowing, dizziness, ear infection, earache, enlarged abdomen, enlarged thyroid gland, eye infection, facial swelling, fast or irregular heartbeat, fatigue, fever, flu-like symptoms, flushing, increased urination, fungal infections, hernia, hiccups, high blood pressure, hives, hot flushes, impotence, increased appetite, indigestion, insomnia, itching, body swelling, liver problems, lymph node problems, menstrual problems, migraine, nausea, nervousness, nosebleed, pain, painful joints and muscles, painful urination, prickly or burning sensation, rash, rectal problems, rigidity, ringing in the ears, runny nose, sensitivity to touch, sinus problems, sleep disorders, sleepiness, sore throat, stomach bleeding, stomach pain, stomach upset, swelling, taste changes, thirst, tremors, urinary tract infection, vaginitis, vertigo, vision changes, vomiting, weakness, weight changes, worsening of arthritis, worsening of asthma, worsening of depression.

The following symptoms are symptoms of an overdose. Notify your Doctor immediately:

Blurred vision, confusion, drowsiness, dry mouth, flushing, headache, nausea, rapid heartbeat, sweating.

Toxicity and adverse reactions:

Nexium comes in delayed-release capsules that should be swallowed whole so be sure to avoid crushing or chewing the capsules.

Amoxil and Biaxin, antibiotics prescribed in conjunction with Nexium for the treatment of ulcers have occasionally been known to cause severe side effects and life-threatening allergic reactions. There's no problem with combining antacids and Nexium.

It is especially important to check with your Doctor before combining Nexium with Diazepam Valium), Digoxin (Lanoxin), Iron salts (Ferro-Sequels) or Ketoconazole (Nizoral).

Oprelvekin [Interleukin-11 - recombinant, rIL-11]

Check with your Doctor if any of the following side effects appear:

Red eyes, weakness, numbness or tingling of hands or feet, skin discoloration, skin rash at place of injection.

261

Always notify your Doctor if any of the following side effects appear:

Fast heartbeat, irregular heartbeat, shortness of breath, sore mouth or tongue, swelling of feet or lower legs, white patches in mouth and/or on tongue, bloody eye, blurred vision, severe redness and peeling of skin.

Your doctor will watch for heart rhythm problems which this medicine may cause.

Oral Mesalamine (Asacol, Pentasa, Mesasal, Salofalk)

Check with your Doctor if any of the following side effects appear:

Mild abdominal or stomach cramps or pain, mild diarrhea, dizziness, mild headache, runny or stuffy nose or sneezing, acne, back or joint pain, gas or flatulence, indigestion, loss of appetite, loss of hair.

Always notify your Doctor if any of the following side effects appear:

Severe abdominal or stomach cramps or pain, bloody diarrhea, fever, severe headache, skin rash and itching, anxiety, severe back pain, blue or pale skin, chest pain, possibly moving to the left arm, neck, or shoulder, chills, fast heartbeat, nausea or vomiting, shortness of breath, swelling of the stomach, unusual tiredness or weakness, yellow eyes or skin.

The following symptoms are symptoms of an overdose. Notify your Doctor immediately:

Confusion, severe or continuing diarrhea, dizziness or lightheadedness, severe drowsiness, fast or deep breathing, severe or continuing headache, hearing loss or continuing ringing or buzzing in ears, continuing nausea or vomiting.

Pancrease (Pancrelipase, Creon, Pancrease MT, Viokase, Ultrase)

Check with your Doctor if any of the following side effects appear:

Stomach and intestinal upset.

Always notify your Doctor if any of the following side effects appear:

Allergic-type reactions.

Immediately notify your Doctor if any of the following side effects appear:

Any signs of an intestinal blockage.

Toxicity and adverse reactions:

Pancrelipase is available in capsule, tablet, and powder forms. Do not change brands or dosage forms of this medication without first checking with your Doctor. The capsules should not be chewed or crushed. If swallowing the capsule is difficult, open the capsule and shake the contents onto a small amount of soft food that does not require chewing, such as applesauce or gelatin, then swallow immediately. Avoid mixing it with alkaline foods, such as ice cream or milk because these can reduce the medication's effect.

Pancrease should be taken with meals and snacks and drink plenty of fluids while you are taking this medication. Do not hold the medication in your mouth as it may irritate the lining. Be careful to avoid inhaling dust from the powdered form as it may irritate the nose, throat, and lungs, and has been known to cause asthma attacks.

Pancrease should not be used if you are sensitive to or have ever had an allergic reaction to pork protein, if you have a recently inflamed pancreas, or if you have a disease of the pancreas that gets worse.

It is especially important that you check with your doctor before combining Pancrease with certain antacids such as Tums and Milk of Magnesia; and certain acid-blocking ulcer medications, such as Pepcid and Zantac

Pepcid (Famotidine, Pepcid AC, Pepcid RPD)

Check with your Doctor if any of the following side effects appear:

Headache.

Always notify your Doctor if any of the following side effects appear:

Abdominal discomfort, acne, agitation, altered taste, anxiety, decreased sex drive, difficulty sleeping, dizziness, dry mouth, dry skin, facial swelling due to fluid retention, fatigue, fever, flushing, hair loss, hallucinations, hives, impotence, itching, loss of appetite, muscle, bone, or joint pain, nausea, prickling, tingling, or pins and needles, rash, ringing in ears, severe allergic reaction, sleepiness, vomiting, weakness, wheezing, jaundice.

Immediately notify your Doctor if any of the following side effects appear:

Breast development in males, changes in behavior, confusion, constipation, depression, diarrhea, grand mal seizures, irregular heartbeat, pounding heartbeat.

Toxicity and adverse reactions:

If you are sensitive to or have ever had an allergic reaction to any H_2 blocker such as Tagamet, Zantac, or Axid, you should not take this medication. If you have stomach cancer, Pepcid may relieve the symptoms without curing the disease and your Doctor must be careful to rule out this possibility.

Use Pepcid with caution if you have severe kidney disease and if you have a condition known as phenylkentonuria, be aware that Pepcid orally isintegrating tablets contain phenylalanine.

You can help avoid heartburn and acid indigestion by not lying down soon after eating, keeping your weight down, stopping smoking, or at least cutting down, avoiding or limiting caffeine, chocolate, fatty foods, alcohol and not eating just before bedtime.

It is especially important that you check with your doctor before combining Pepcid with Itraconazole (Sporanox) or Ketoconazole (Nizoral).

Prednisone (Deltasone)

Check with your Doctor if any of the following side effects appear:

> Increased appetite, indigestion, nervousness or restlessness, darkening or lightening of skin color, dizziness or lightheadedness, flushing of face or cheeks, hiccups, increased joint pain (after injection into a joint), increased sweating, sensation of spinning.

Always notify your Doctor if any of the following side effects appear:

> Decreased or blurred vision, frequent urination, increased thirst, sudden blindness (when injected in the head or neck area), burning, numbness, pain, or tingling at or near place of injection, confusion, excitement, false sense of well-being, hallucinations, depression, mistaken feelings of self-importance or being mistreated, sudden and wide mood swings, redness, swelling, or other sign of allergy or infection at place of injection, restlessness, skin rash or hives.

The following list of side effects may occur when this drug is used for a prolonged period of time. Check with your Doctor if any of the following side effects appear:

> Abdominal pain, acne, bloody or black, tarry stools, changes in vision, eye pain, filling or rounding out

of the face, headache, irregular heartbeat, menstrual problems, muscle cramps, muscle pain or weakness, nausea, pain in arms, back, hips, legs, ribs, or shoulders, pitting, scarring, or depression of skin at place of injection, reddish purple lines on arms, face, groin, legs, or trunk, redness of eyes, sensitivity of eyes to light, stunting of growth in children, swelling of feet or lower legs, tearing of eyes, thin, shiny skin, trouble in sleeping, unusual bruising, unusual increase in hair growth, unusual tiredness or weakness, vomiting, rapid weight gain, wounds that will not heal.

Important Note

Corticosteroids may lower your resistance to infections. Any infection you get may be harder to treat. Check with your doctor as soon as possible if you notice any possible signs of an infection, such as sore throat, fever, sneezing, or coughing.

After stopping this medicine, the body may need time to adjust. The length of time this takes depends on the amount of Prednisone you have taken and how long it was used. After taking large doses of this medicine for a long period of time, it may take up to a full year for your body to adjust. During this time, immediately check with your doctor if any of the following side effects appear:

Abdominal, stomach, or back pain, dizziness, fainting, fever, continuing loss of appetite, muscle or joint pain, nausea, reappearance of disease symptoms shortness of breath, unexplained headaches, unusual tiredness, frequent or continuing weakness, vomiting, rapid weight loss.

267

Patients on long-term Prednisone therapy should wear or carry identification.

Prednisone should also be taken with caution if you have diverticulitis, high blood pressure, kidney disorder, myasthenia gravis, which is a muscle-weakness disorder, osteoporosis, peptic ulcer, Crohn's disease or ulcerative colitis.

Diseases such as chickenpox or measles can be very serious or even fatal in both children and adults who are taking this drug. Try to avoid exposure to these diseases.

Check with your Doctor before combining Prednisone with Amphotericin B (Fungizone), Coumadin, Carbamazepine (Tegretol), Estrogen drugs such as Premarin, Ketoconazole (Nizoral), Oral contraceptives, Phenobarbital, Donnatal, Phenytoin (Dilantin), Lasix, Rifampin (Rifadin), Troleandomycin (Tao).

Prevacid (Lansoprazole)

Check with your Doctor if any of the following side effects appear:

Abdominal pain, acne, nausea, hiccups, high blood pressure, high or low blood sugar, hives, impotence, increased appetite, increased salivation, indigestion, itching, loss of appetite, low blood pressure, memory loss, menstrual problems, muscle, bone, or joint pain, nervousness, prickling, tingling, or pins and needles, rash, taste alteration, thirst, visual disturbances, vomiting blood, weakness, weight gain or loss, wheezing, yeast infection.

Always notify your Doctor if any of the following side effects appear:

Diarrhea, asthma, bad breath, belching, black or discolored stools, blood in the urine, constipation, cough, decreased sex drive, dry mouth, ear infection, eye pain, fainting, fever, fluid retention, "flu-like" symptoms, flushing, gallstones, gas, general feeling of illness, gout, hair loss, hallucinations.

Immediately notify your Doctor if any of the following side effects appear:

Abnormal thinking, aggravation of hostility, agitation, anemia, anxiety, apathy, arthritis, breast development in males, breast enlargement, breast tenderness, bronchitis, chest pain (including severe pain), colitis, confusion, coughing up blood, deafness, depression, diabetes, difficult or labored breathing, difficulty swallowing, dizziness, heart attack, infection, inflammation of the esophagus or mouth, inflammation of the stomach lining, kidney problems, kidney stones, nosebleeds, paralysis, pneumonia, rectal hemorrhage, rectal and bladder spasms, ringing in ears, shock, sore throat, stomach and intestinal hemorrhage, stroke, throbbing heartbeat, thyroid problems.

Toxicity and adverse reactions:

Prevacid should be taken before meals. If you have trouble swallowing the capsules, open them and sprinkle the granules on a tablespoon of applesauce;

swallow immediately. Do not chew or crush the granules.

If you are taking antacids for pain, you may continue to do so. You also may continue to take Carafate, but take your dose of Prevacid at least 30 minutes prior to the Carafate.

This medication should not be used for long-term therapy of duodenal ulcer or erosive esophagitis and if you have liver disease, be sure your Doctor knows about it because Prevacid should be used cautiously.

It is especially important to check with your doctor before combining Prevacid with Ampicillin, Digoxin (Lanoxin), Iron salts (Ferro-Sequels, Ferro-Sulfate), Ketoconazole (Nizoral), Sucralfate (Carafate), Theophylline (Theo-Dur

Prilosec (Omeprazole)

Check with your Doctor if any of the following side effects appear:

Abdominal pain, diarrhea, headache, nausea, vomiting.

Always notify your Doctor if any of the following side effects appear:

Abdominal swelling, abnormal dreams, apathy, back pain, discolored feces, dizziness, dry mouth, dry skin, fatigue, fever, fluid retention and swelling, gas, general feeling of illness, hair loss, hallucinations, hepatitis, high blood pressure, hives, irritable colon, itching, joint and leg pain, loss of appetite, muscle

270

cramps and pain, nervousness, nosebleeds, taste distortion, tingling or pins and needles, throat pain, tremors, upper respiratory infection, urinary tract infection, vertigo, weakness, weight gain, yellow eyes and skin.

Immediately notify your Doctor if any of the following side effects appear:

Aggression, anemia, anxiety, breast development in males, blood in urine, changes in liver function, chest pain, confusion, constipation, cough, depression, difficulty sleeping, fluttery heartbeat, frequent urination, low blood sugar, pain, pain in testicles, rapid heartbeat, rash, ringing in ears, skin inflammation, sleepiness, slow heartbeat, stomach tumors.

The following symptoms are symptoms of an overdose. Notify your Doctor immediately:

Blurred vision, confusion, drowsiness, dry mouth, flushing, headache, nausea, rapid heartbeat, sweating.

Toxicity and adverse reactions:

Prilosec's healing effect can mask the signs of stomach cancer and your Doctor should be careful to rule out this possibility.

The capsule should be swallowed whole and should not be opened, chewed, or crushed.

It may take several days for Prilosec to begin relieving stomach pain and long-term use of this medication can cause severe stomach inflammation and you should avoid excessive amounts of caffeine while taking this drug.

When taken with Biaxin, side effects also may include flu symptoms, nasal inflammation, sore throat, taste alteration, tongue discoloration. When taken with Amoxicillin and Biaxin, side effects also may include diarrhea, headache, taste alteration.

It is especially important to check with your doctor before combining Prilosec with Ampicillin-containing drugs such as Unasyn, Cyclosporine (Sandimmune, Neoral), Diazepam (Valium), Disulfiram (Antabuse), Iron, Ketoconazole (Nizoral), Phenytoin (Dilantin), Coumadin. When taking the Prilosec/Biaxin combination treatment, it's best to avoid the hay-fever remedy Hismanal.

Psorcon (Diflorasone diacetate)

Check with your Doctor if any of the following side effects appear:

Burning, dryness, eruptions resembling acne, excessive discoloring of the skin, excessive growth of hair, inflammation of hair follicles, inflammation around the mouth, irritation, itching, prickly heat, secondary infection, severe inflammation of the skin, softening of the skin, stretch marks, stretching or thinning of the skin.

Toxicity and adverse reactions:

Psorcon is available in ointment and cream forms, and in emollient ointment and cream.

Psorcon is for use only on the skin so be very careful to keep it out of your eyes.

If you are sensitive to or have ever had an allergic reaction to Diflorasone diacetate or other antifungal or Corticosteriod medications, you should not take this medication.

Your Doctor will limit the use of Psorcon for your child to the least amount that is effective because long-term treatment may interfere with the growth and development of children.

Rectal Mesalamine (Rowasa, Salofalk)

Check with your Doctor if any of the following side effects appear:

Mild abdominal or stomach cramps or pain, gas or flatulence, mild headache, nausea, loss of hair.

Always notify your Doctor if any of the following side effects appear:

Severe abdominal or stomach cramps or pain, anxiety, severe back pain, bloody diarrhea, blue or pale skin, chest pain, possibly moving to the left arm, neck, or shoulder, chills, fast heartbeat, fever, severe headache, nausea or vomiting, rectal irritation, shortness of breath, skin rash, swelling of the stomach, unusual tiredness or weakness, yellow eyes or skin.

Reglan (Metoclopramide hydrochloride)

Check with your Doctor if any of the following side effects appear:

Drowsiness, fatigue, restlessness.

Always notify your Doctor if any of the following side effects appear:

Diarrhea, dizziness, fluid retention, frequent urination, hallucinations, headache, high or low blood pressure, hives, insomnia, menstrual irregularities, nausea, rash, jaundice.

Immediately notify your Doctor if any of the following side effects appear:

Breast development in males, confusion, congestive heart failure, continual discharge of milk from the breasts, depression, high fever, impotence, inability to hold urine, rapid or slow heartbeat, rigid muscles, slow movement, swollen tongue or throat, tremor, vision problems, wheezing.

The following symptoms are symptoms of an overdose. Notify your Doctor immediately:

Disorientation, drowsiness, involuntary movements.

Toxicity and adverse reactions:

Reglan may cause symptoms similar to those of Parkinson's disease. If you have Parkinson's disease, you should be given Reglan cautiously or not at all, since the drug may make your Parkinson's symptoms worse.

Especially in older people, Reglan may produce Tardive dyskinesia, which is a syndrome of jerky or writhing involuntary movements, particularly of the tongue, face, mouth, or jaw. In children and adults under 30, Reglan may cause involuntary movements of the arms and legs, and sometimes loud or labored breathing, usually in the first day or two of treatment. Reglan is not recommended for patients under 18 years of age.

You should not take Reglan, if you have obstruction, perforation, or hemorrhage of the stomach or small bowel that might be aggravated by increased stomach and small-bowel movement; if you have Pheochromocytoma, which is a nonmalignant tumor that causes hypertension as it could trigger a dangerous jump in blood pressure; if you have epilepsy as it could increase the frequency and severity of seizures.

It is especially important to check with your doctor before combining Reglan with Acetaminophen, Alcoholic beverages, Bentyl, Pro-Banthine, Tagamet, Cyclosporine Digoxin (Lanoxin), Insulin, Nardil, Parnate, Levodopa (Sinemet), Percocet, Demerol, Dalmane, Halcion, Restoril, Tetracycline, Valium and Xanax.

Temovate (Clobetasol propionate, Cormax)

Check with your Doctor if any of the following side effects appear:

Burning, cracking/fissuring, irritation, itching, numbness of fingers, patches, reddened skin, shrinking of the skin, stinging, acne, allergic skin inflammation, dryness, excessive hair growth, infection, inflammation around the mouth, loss of skin color, prickly heat, skin softening, streaking.

Always notify your Doctor if any of the following side effects appear:

Eye irritation, hair loss, headache, inflammation, itching, tenderness and/or tightness of the scalp (these side effects are usually found with the scalp application)

Toxicity and adverse reactions:

Temovate and Cormax relieve the itching and inflammation of moderate to severe skin conditions. The scalp application is used for short-term treatment of scalp conditions while the cream, ointment, emollient cream, and gel are used for short-term treatment of skin conditions on the body.

These products contain a steroid medication for external use only.

Do not use this medication more often or for a longer time than ordered which is usually no more than 2 weeks. Temovate is for use only on the skin so be very careful to keep it out of your eyes and if it does get into your eyes, flush your eyes with a lot of water.

Do not use this medications near an open flame.

All forms of Temovate should be avoided if you are sensitive to or have ever had an allergic reaction to Clobetasol propionate or other Corticosteroids or their ingredients. Do not use the scalp application if you have a scalp infection.

Temovate is a strong Corticosteroid that can be absorbed into the bloodstream. It has caused Cushing's syndrome, emotional disturbances, high blood pressure, weight gain, and, in women, abnormal growth of facial and body hair. It has also affected changes in blood sugar.

Tetracycline (Achromycin V, Sumycin)

Check with your Doctor if any of the following side effects appear:

Genital irritation and discharge, skin problem becomes worse

Notify your Doctor if any of the following side effects appear:

Severe headaches, yeast infection

Toxicity and adverse reactions:

Tetracycline only suppress the conditions, they do not cure them. Therefore these antibiotics need to be continued until the disease runs it course, often months or years. Long term treatment with Tetracycline is remarkably safe with over 30 years experience with the medication.

Tetracycline should be stored in a cool place out of direct sunlight. Outdated capsules or tablets should not be taken as they may cause kidney damage.

Tetracycline must not be taken during pregnancy or while breast-feeding. Children under twelve years old should not take this medication because it discolors growing teeth.

Tetracycline should be taken with a glass of water on an empty stomach, half an hour before or two hours after meals because food prevents absorption of the medication into the bloodstream. Some people find this inconvenient, and others get indigestion unless it is taken with food.

Tetracycline may make the skin more sensitive to sunlight. This effect depends on the variety of Tetracycline and the amount taken. If unexpected sunburn does occur, take the medication in the evening and avoid excessive sun exposure.

Thalidomide (Thalomid)

Check with your Doctor if any of the following side effects appear:

Constipation, diarrhea, dizziness, drowsiness, nausea, stomach pain, dryness of mouth, dry skin, headache, increased appetite, mood changes, swelling in the legs.

Immediately notify your Doctor if any of the following side effects appear:

Muscle weakness, tingling, burning, numbness, or pain in the hands, arms, feet, or legs, blood in urine, decreased urination, fever, alone or with chills and sore throat, irregular heartbeat, low blood pressure, skin rash.

Topicort (Desoximetasone)

Check with your Doctor if any of the following side effects appear:

Acne-like pimples, blistering, burning of the skin, dryness, excessive growth of hair, infection, inflammation of the hair follicles, irritation, itching, loss of skin pigmentation, prickly heat, skin inflammation around the mouth, rash, redness, softening of the skin, stretch marks on the skin, thinning of the skin.

Toxicity and adverse reactions:

Do not use Topicort if you are sensitive to it or have ever had an allergic reaction to any of its ingredients.

Long-term use of steroids such as Topicort may interfere with the growth and development of children. They may also develop headaches, or bulging at the top of the head. This drug is not recommended for children under 10.

Large doses of steroids such as Topicort applied over a large area or for a long time, especially when the treated area is covered, can cause increases in blood sugar and Cushing's syndrome.

Tridesilon (Desonide, DesOwen)

Check with your Doctor if any of the following side effects appear:

Acne, additional infections, allergic reactions of the skin, burning and stinging, dryness, excessive hair growth, irritation, itching, loss of skin color, prickly heat, rash, scaly skin, inflammation around the mouth, skin loss, skin peeling or redness, skin softening, stretch marks, worsening of the condition.

Side effects that may occur in children may include delayed weight gain, headaches, slowed growth.

Always notify your Doctor if any of the following side effects appear:

Increases in blood sugar or sugar in the urine, Cushing's syndrome, any effect on the adrenal gland, pituitary, and hypothalamus; irritation of the skin or your conditions has lasted more than two weeks.

Toxicity and adverse reactions:

Tridesilon is for use only on the skin so be very careful to keep it out of your eyes.

Safety and effectiveness of DesOwen in children have not been established.

With overuse or misuse of Tridesilon, too much medicine can enter the body, causing increases in blood sugar and Cushing's syndrome.

Zantac

Check with your Doctor if any of the following side effects appear:

Abdominal discomfort and pain, agitation, changes in blood count or anemia, changes in liver function, constipation, depression, diarrhea, difficulty sleeping, dizziness, hair loss, hallucinations, heart block, hepatitis, hypersensitivity reactions, inflammation of the pancreas, involuntary movements, irregular heartbeat, jaundice, joint pain, muscle pain, nausea and vomiting, rapid heartbeat, rash, reduced white blood cells, reversible mental confusion, sleepiness, slow heartbeat, vague feeling of bodily discomfort or vertigo.

Always notify your Doctor if any of the following side effects appear:

Severe headache.

Immediately notify your Doctor if any of the following side effects appear:

Abnormal manner of walking, low blood pressure, and exaggerated side effect of other symptoms. These symptoms are symptoms of an overdose.

Toxicity and adverse reactions:

Take this medication exactly as prescribed by your doctor. Make sure you follow the diet your doctor recommends. Dissolve "Efferdose" tablets and granules in 6 to 8 ounces of water before taking them. You can take an antacid for pain while you are taking Zantac.

If you have kidney or liver disease, this drug should be used with caution. If you have phenylketonuria, you should be aware that the "Efferdose" tablets and granules contain phenylalanine.

It is especially important to check with your Doctor before combining Zantac with Alcohol, blood-thinning drugs such as Coumadin, Diazepam (Valium), Diltiazem (Cardizem), Enoxacin (Penetrex), Glipizide (Glucotrol), Glyburide (DiaBeta, Micronase), Itraconazole (Sporanox), Ketoconazole (Nizoral), Metformin (Glucophage), Nifedipine (Procardia), Phenytoin (Dilantin), Procainamide (Procan SR), Sucralfate (Carafate), Theophylline (Theo-Dur), Triazolam (Halcion).

Zyloprim (Allopurinol)

Check with your Doctor if any of the following side effects appear:

Abdominal pain, bruising, chills, fever, hair loss, headache, hepatitis, hives, indigestion, itching, joint pain, kidney failure, loosening of nails, muscle disease, nosebleed, severe blisters or bleeding on the lips, eyes, or nose, sleepiness, stomach inflammation, taste loss or change, tingling or pins and needles, unusual bleeding, vomiting, yellowing of skin and eyes more commonly called jaundice.

Always notify your Doctor if any of the following side effects appear:

Acute attack of gout, diarrhea, nausea.

Immediately notify your Doctor if any of the following side effects appear:

A rash of any kind or any other sign of an allergic reaction.

Toxicity and adverse reactions:

It is important to note that Zyloprim will not stop a gout attack that is already underway. To help prevent attacks of gout, you should avoid beer, wine, and purine-rich foods such as anchovies, sardines, liver, kidneys, lentils, and sweetbreads.

If you have been taking Colchicine or any other anti-inflammatory medication such as Anaprox or Indocin to relieve your gout, your Doctor will probably want you to continue taking this medication while your Zyloprim dosage is being adjusted. When you have had no attacks of gout for several months, you may be able to stop taking these other medications.

If you have been taking medications that promote the excretion of uric acid in the urine, such as Probenecid (Benemid) or Sulfinpyrazone (Anturane), to prevent attacks of gout, your Doctor will probably reduce or stop your dosage of these medications while increasing your dosage of Zyloprim.

You should avoid taking large doses of vitamin C because of the increased possibility of kidney stone formation. While taking Zyloprim you should drink 10 to 12 glasses of water per day.

Zyloprim is also used to manage the increased uric acid levels in the blood of people with certain cancers such as leukemia. It is also prescribed to manage some types of kidney stones.

A kidney problem may turn a normal dose of Zyloprim into an overdose. If you have a kidney disease, diabetes or high blood pressure, your Doctor should prescribe Zyloprim cautiously and order periodic blood and urine tests to assess your kidney function.

It is especially important to check with your doctor before combining Zyloprim with Amoxicillin (Amoxil, Trimox, Wymox), Ampicillin (Omnipen, Principen), Azathioprine (Imuran), Coumadin, Cyclosporine (Sandimmune, Neoral), Diabinese and Orinase, Mercaptopurine (Purinethol), Probenecid (Benemid, ColBENEMID), Sulfinpyrazone (Anturane), Theophylline (Theo-Dur, Slo-Phyllin), thiazide diuretics such as HydroDIURIL and Diuril.

Chapter 14

Non-Steroidal
Anti-Inflammatory Drugs

Non-Steroidal Anti-Inflammatory Drugs, (NSAID's) are found in almost every medicine cabinet across America and are so numerous that in drugstores and grocery stores they usually have their own aisle. People use NSAID's for headaches, muscle pain, arthritis pain, menstrual cramps and many other every day aches and pains.

Many patients with Crohn's disease experience pain on a daily basis due to related conditions such as arthritis or drug side effects such as headaches. Many gastroenterologists however, recommend that their patients avoid taking NSAID's because they are known to have an adverse effect on Crohn's disease and ulcerative colitis.

NSAID's can contribute to ulcers in both the stomach and the first part of the small intestine even in people without Crohn's disease. They can also cause inflammation and worsen bleeding in the small intestine and these drugs have been known to knock some people with Crohn's disease out of remission. Patients with Crohn's disease should consult with their gastroenterologist before taking any of these meds, even those available over the counter.

There is some good news for those who have Crohn's disease and are looking for over the counter pain relief. Acetaminophen, which is sold under many brand names including Tylenol®, is not an NSAID and may be safe for people with Crohn's disease. Still, you should consult with your doctor before taking this drug.

Following is a list of NSAID's available by prescription or over the counter. This is by no means a comprehensive or exhaustive list. You should consult your pharmacist for concerns about specific drugs.

NSAID's
Brand Names and Generic Equivalents

Brand Name	Generic Equivalent
Advil, Excedrin IB, Genpril, Haltran, Ibuprin, Ibuprohm, Ibu-Tab, Midrin 200, Medipren, Midol IB, Motrin, Nuprin, Pamprin-IB, Rufen, Trendar, Advil Liqui-Gels	Ibuprofen
Aleve, Anaprox, Naprosyn Sodium	Naproxen
Amigesic, Anaflex 750, Marthritic, Mono-Gesic, Salflex, Salsitab, Disalcid	Salsalate
Anacin, Bayer, Bufferin, Ecotrin salicylate	Choline
Ansaid, Froben, Froben SR	Flurbiprofen
Apo-Keto, Orudis, Oruvail, Rhodis	Ketoprofen
Apo-Sulin, Clinoril, Novo-Sundac	Sulindac
Aspergum, Genuine Bayer, Bayer Childrens, Bufferin, Easprin, Ecotrin, Empirin, Genprin, Halfprin, Magnaprin, ZORprin	Aspirin
Butazolidin	Phenylbutazone
Cataflam, Voltaren	Diclofenac

DayPro	Oxaprozin
Dolobid	Diflunisal
Feldene, Novo-Pirocam, Nu-Pirox	Piroxicam
Indocin SR, Indocid, Indocid SR, Novo-Methacin	Indomethacin
Lodine, Lodine XL	Etodolac
Meclomen	Meclofenamate Sodium
Mobic	Meloxicam
Fenoprofen	Calcium
Ponstan, Ponstel	Mefenamic Acid
Relafen	Nabumetone
Tolmetin	Sodium

Chapter 15

Vitamins and Supplements

As most of you has probably read or heard in recent years, many nutritionists applaud the virtues of low-fat diets. However some fat intake is necessary for the body to absorb certain vitamins such as A, D, E, and K.

The use of vitamins and minerals in the body is a complex process, with many nutrients depending on others to facilitate the absorption and use by the body. If the body is not receiving even one nutrient it needs, the end result is a chain reaction affecting many other vitamins and minerals. There are three main factors that contribute to vitamin and mineral deficiencies in people with Crohn's disease.

The first factor is inflammation in the small and/or large intestine. Fat is absorbed in the small intestine and unfortunately, people who have Crohn's disease or ulcerative colitis; fat absorption is a particular problem. Because of this, some nutrients are not fully absorbed. Additionally, a small intestine or colon that has undergone surgery to remove diseased sections could severely impair the ability to absorb fat and the fat-soluble vitamins.

The second factor is the often-restricted diets that people with Crohn's disease or ulcerative colitis follow to curb or prevent symptoms. Nausea, diarrhea, and vomiting make getting a balanced diet an almost impossible task.

The third factor is a result of treatment programs that often include many different types of medications. Some of these medications can inhibit the absorption of nutrients, or cause them to be lost from the body.

There are two types of Vitamins. They are Fat Soluble and Water Soluble. Fat Soluble Vitamins include Vitamins A, D, E and K. Water Soluble Vitamins include Vitamins B1, B2, B3, B5, B6, B12, Vitamin C, Folate, Choline, Inositol, PABA (Para-aminobenzoic Acid) and Biotin.

There are two types of Minerals. Major Minerals includes Calcium, Phosphorus, Magnesium, Sodium, Chloride, Potassium and Sulfur. Trace Minerals include Iodine, Iron, Zinc, Copper, Fluoride, Selenium, Chromium, Molybdenum, Manganese and Cobalt.

There are two types of Amino Acids. They are Essential Amino Acids that include Histidine, Isoleucine, Leucine, Lysine, Methionine, Phenylalanine, Threonine, Tryptophan and Valine. Non-essential Amino Acids include Alanine, Arginine, Asparagine, Aspartic acid, Cysteine, Glutamic acid, Glutamine, Glycine, Proline, Serine and Tyrosine.

The following list of Vitamins / Supplements is included for your reference. Before starting any program that include the taking of any of these supplements; make sure that you discuss the program with your doctor.

Vitamin A (Retinol / Beta-carotene)

Recommended Daily Allowance:

1,000 mg for males
800 mg for females
1,300 for pregnancy (2nd and 3rd Trimester)

Type: Fat Soluble Vitamin

Some Food Sources for Vitamin A:

Apricots, Papaya, Beef liver, Pumpkin, Broccoli, Pork liver, Cantaloupe, Spinach, Carrot, Sweet potato, Chicken liver, Winter squash, Mango, Dairy products.

Side Effects and Toxicity:

Signs of toxicity are usually noticed after 6 - 8 months of ingestion. Toxicity from Vitamin A include red blood cell damage, abdominal cramps, blurred vision, irritability, bone pain, loss of appetite, diarrhea, nosebleeds, growth retardation, hair loss, skin rashes, dry skin, liver disease, nausea, vomiting, headache and increased cerebrospinal pressure.

When taken in early pregnancy Vitamin A may increase risk of birth defects.

Palmitate, the synthetic form, is most toxic.

Patients with liver dysfunction from alcohol, drugs, hepatic diseases, elderly, protein calorie malnutrition, have increased susceptibility to vitamin A toxicity.

Vitamin D (Cholecalciferol / Ergocalciferol)

Recommended Daily Allowance:

5 mg
7.5 mg during pregnancy / lactation

Type: Fat Soluble Vitamin

Some Food Sources for Vitamin D:

Beef, Lamb, Butter, Mackerel, Chicken, Pork, Cream, Sunshine (20 minutes per day), Egg yolk, Salmon, Fortified Milk, Shrimp, Halibut, Sardines, Herring.

Side Effects and Toxicity:

There are reports that 25mg - 30mg per day in children may produce symptoms of toxicity such as calcification of soft tissues such as the kidneys, lungs or the inner ear membrane.

When taking Vitamin D, you may experience constipation or diarrhea, headaches, nausea, raised blood calcium, weight loss, irritability, weakness, kidney stones, mental retardation, physical retardation, hypercalcemia, hypercalciuria, soft tissue calcifications.

Vitamin E (Tocopherol / Tocotrienol)

Recommended Daily Allowance:

15 mg

Type: Fat Soluble Vitamin

Some Food Sources for Vitamin E:

Almonds, Pecans, Cod liver oil, Safflower oil, Corn oil, Sunflower oil, Flax oil, Sunflower seeds, Hazelnuts, Wheat germ, Peanuts, Wild purslane (leafy veggie), Peanut butter

Side Effects and Toxicity:

For Patients with diabetes and rheumatic heart disease, start with low doses (8 -10 mg / day) and build slowly.

Taken in doses greater than 20 mg / day, you may experience diarrhea, fainting, flatulence, headache, heart palpitations, hypertension, increased triglycerides or nausea. All of these symptoms are completely reversible with decreased dosage.

There is no well-documented toxicity of vitamin E other than general discomfort and this symptom is rare.

Vitamin K (Quinones)

Recommended Daily Allowance:

70 - 80 mg for males
60 - 65 mg for females

Type: Fat Soluble Vitamin

Some Food Sources for Vitamin K:

Asparagus, Peaches, Beef liver, Peas, Broccoli,
cooked, Cabbage, Spinach, Cheese, Green beans,
Watercress, Green tea, Lettuce

Non-Food Source:

Intestinal flora - bacterial synthesis in the digestive
tract.

Side Effects and Toxicity:

Vitamin K is generally well tolerated at usual doses;
however, it may produce hemolytic anemia and
jaundice if taken in large doses.

Vitamin C (Ascorbic Acid)

Recommended Daily Allowance:

90 mg for males
75 mg for females

Type: Water Soluble Vitamin

Some Food Sources for Vitamin C:

Broccoli, Mango, Brussels sprouts, Orange juice,
Cantaloupe, Papaya, Green peppers, Potatoes,
Grapefruit, Strawberries, Grapefruit juice, Tomato
juice, Guava, Watermelon, Kiwi fruit

Side Effects and Toxicity:

When taking Vitamin C, cholesterol tests may be affected; you may give false negative test for glucose in urine and may give false negative test for occult blood in urine. You may have nausea, diarrhea, red blood cell damage, nosebleeds, and abdominal cramps. There is an increased absorption of iron and when taken in large doses, intestinal gas and diarrhea may be experienced.

Multivitamins (Centrum, Theragran, Vi-Daylin)

Multivitamins are nutritional supplements for people whose diet may be deficient in certain vitamins and minerals. You may need a supplement if you are on a special diet, or don't eat the right foods. A supplement may also be necessary if you are a strict vegetarian, take medications that prevent the body from using certain nutrients, or have an illness that affects your appetite. In addition, special formulas are available for use during pregnancy.

Vitamin/mineral supplements come in a wide range of formulations. Three of the most widely used are Centrum, Theragran, and Vi-Daylin. Each of these brands offers a variety of formulas tailored to the needs of different groups.

Centrum is a multivitamin/multimineral supplement that includes all antioxidants, the vitamins that strengthen the body's natural defenses against cell damage. *Centrum Silver* contains higher strengths of the vitamins that people 50 years of age or older need the most. *Centrum, Jr.*, formulations are geared to children's needs.

295

Theragran is a multivitamin supplement. *Theragran-M* adds minerals to the formulation. *Theragran Stress Formula* contains higher strengths of the B vitamins that may be needed for people under stress, plus extra vitamin C.

Vi-Daylin is a multivitamin supplement; *Vi-Daylin + Iron* is a multivitamin plus iron, which may be needed by women who have heavy menstrual periods. Some Vi-Daylin formulations also contain fluoride. *Vi-Daylin drops* are given to infants and young children.

Do not use supplements as a replacement for a diet rich in essential vitamins and minerals. Food contains many important ingredients not available in supplements. If you have any serious chronic medical conditions check with your Doctor before starting on a multivitamin supplement because you may have special requirements. If your multivitamin supplement contains Fluoride, check with your Doctor because you should not use it if your drinking water contains more than 0.7 parts per million of Fluoride.

The usual dose for an adult is 1 tablet, teaspoonful, or tablespoonful daily according to package instructions, or as directed by your Doctor. The usual dose of children's formulations is 1 tablet, teaspoonful, or dropper full daily or as directed by your Doctor. Younger children may require only half this dose.

Megadoses of some vitamins and minerals can be harmful when taken for extended periods. If you have unexplained symptoms and suspect an overdose, check with Doctor.

Vitamin B - Complex

The "B" family of vitamins is a water-soluble vitamin. These vitamins are used as enzymes for a variety of biochemical reactions in almost all parts of the body. They are essential for building and maintaining healthy nerves, skin, hair, eyes, liver, mouth, and the entire gastrointestinal tract. B vitamins provide energy by assisting in the metabolism of carbohydrates, fats, and proteins. They are associated with a healthy immune system and the prevention of aging and are depleted by stress.

The B Vitamin family includes:

Vitamin B1   (Thiamin)
Vitamin B12 (Cobalamin)
Vitamin B2   (Riboflavin)
Biotin
Vitamin B3   (Niacin)
Folate
Vitamin B5   (Pantothenic Acid)
Choline (Lecithin)
Vitamin B6   (Pyridoxine)
Inositol
PABA (Para-aminobenzoic Acid)

Vitamin B1 (Thiamin)

Recommended Daily Allowance:

1.0 - 1.5 mg

Type: Water Soluble Vitamin

Some Food Sources for Vitamin B-1:

Beef kidney, Rolled oats, Beef liver, Dark rye,
Brewer's yeast, Soy flour, brown rice, Soybeans,
Chick peas, Sunflower seeds, Kidney beans, Wheat
germ, Navy beans, Whole wheat flour, Pork, Poultry

Side Effects and Toxicity:

Although rare, side effects include rapid pulse,
weakness, headaches, insomnia, irritability. High
doses of Vitamin B1 may cause Vitamin B6 or
Magnesium deficiencies.

Vitamin B2 (Riboflavin)

Recommended Daily Allowance:

1.7 mg for males
1.3 mg for females
    additional 0.3 mg during pregnancy
    additional 0.5 mg during lactation

Type: Water Soluble Vitamin

Some Food Sources for Vitamin B2:

Almonds, Calf heart, Beef heart, Camembert cheese,
Beef kidney, Chicken liver, Beef liver, Milk,
Brewer's yeast, Wild rice, Brie cheese, Roquefort
cheese, Broccoli, Yogurt, Breads, Cereals, Eggs

Side Effects and Toxicity:

There are no known toxicity effects associated with Vitamin B2.

Vitamin B3 (Niacin / Nicotinic acid / Nicotinamide)

Recommended daily allowance

13 - 18 NE (Niacin Equivelants)
    additional 2 NE / day during pregnancy
    additional 5 NE / day during lactation

Type: Water Soluble Vitamin

Some Food Sources for Vitamin B3:

Beef, Cod, Beef kidney, Halibut, Beef liver, Peanuts, Brewer's yeast, Salmon steak, Brown rice, Sunflower seeds, Chicken, Swordfish, Chicken liver, Tuna, Cereals, Fortified Milk

Side Effects and Toxicity:

Nausea is first sign of toxicity with Vitamin B3. Flushing may occur when taking Vitamin B3, so it is recommended that this vitamin be taken with food. Side effects include gastritis, increases uric acid levels, low blood pressure, skin flushing, headaches, ulcer irritation, hepatic / liver abnormalities, nausea and this vitamin will reactivate peptic ulcers.

Liver enzymes should be monitored during Vitamin B3 therapy. If enzymes are elevated you should cut back on the dosage.

Vitamin B5 (Pantothenic Acid)

Recommended Daily Allowance:

4 - 7 mg

Type: Water Soluble Vitamin

Some Food Sources for Vitamin B5:

Beef liver, Chicken, Chicken liver, Hard boiled egg, Beef kidney, Brown rice, Turkey, Sweet corn, Brewer's yeast, Beef, Peas, Sweet potato, Peanuts, Cashews

Side Effects and Toxicity:

Some adverse effects of taking Vitamin B5 in large doses will be diarrhea. This will stop once the vitamin is stopped.

Vitamin B6 (Pyridoxine hydrochloride / pyridoxal / pyridoxamine)

Recommended Daily Allowance:

2 mg - 2.2 mg
2.6 mg - 2.7 mg for pregnancy / lactation

Type: Water Soluble Vitamin

Some Food Sources for Vitamin B6:

100% bran cereal, Salmon, Sunflower seeds, Avocado, Tomato juice, Banana, Trout, Beef liver, Turkey, Watermelon, Chicken, Pork loin chop

300

Side Effects and Toxicity:

Some side effects are numbness and tingling in the extremities if 2 - 3 gm per day are taken over a few months. Doses larger than 50mg / day may suppress lactation. Lower does may cause insomnia or anxiety that may be prevented by taking magnesium. Other more common side effects are depression, fatigue, irritability, and headaches.

These effects usually disappear after Vitamin B6 is discontinued.

Vitamin B12 (Cobalamin)

Recommended Daily Allowance

2 mg
2.2 mg during pregnancy
2.6 mg during lactation

(Strict vegetarians should consult a physician before taking B12 supplements)

Type: Water Soluble Vitamin

Some Food Sources for Vitamin B12:

Beef, Halibut, Beef liver, Lamb, Brewer's yeast, Lobster, Cheese, Milk, Chicken, Salmon steak, Clams, Tuna, Eggs

Side Effects and Toxicity:

There are no known side effects or toxicity associated with Vitamin B12.

Folate (Folic Acid / Folacin)

Recommended Daily Allowance

400 mg
600 mg during pregnancy
500 mg during lactation

Type: Water Soluble Vitamin

Some Food Sources for Folate:

Beef liver, Cantaloupe, Beets, Chicken liver, Black-eyed peas, Egg yolk, Brewer's yeast, Orange juice, Broccoli, Romaine lettuce, Brussels sprouts, Wheat bran, Breads, Cereals

Side Effects and Toxicity:

Some side effects of Folate are that it may interfere with the laboratory diagnosis of pernicious anemia and large doses may promote seizures in preexisting epilepsy. More common side effects are insomnia, irritability, diarrhea, and Folate may make a Vitamin B12 deficiency.

Biotin (Vitamin H / Coenzyme R)

Recommended Daily Allowance

30 - 100 mg

Type: Water Soluble Vitamin

Some Food Sources for Biotin:

Calf liver, Halibut, Camembert cheese, Milk, Chicken, Lamb kidney, Chicken liver, Rolled oats, Cod, Salmon steak, Hard boiled egg, Tuna, Haddock

Side Effects and Toxicity:

There are no known adverse effects or toxicity associated with Biotin.

Choline (Lecithin)

Recommended Daily Allowance:

300 - 900 mg

Type: Water Soluble Vitamin

Some Food Sources for Choline:

Egg yolk, Legumes, Milk, Muscle meats, Organ meats, Whole-grain cereals, Fish

Side Effects and Toxicity:

Some adverse effects and toxicity of Choline are depression, diarrhea, dizziness, fishy odor and nausea.

Inositol (Vitamin B8 / Phytic Acid / Inositol Hexaphosphate / IP6 / Myoinositol)

Recommended Daily Allowance:

500 mg

Type: Water Soluble Vitamin

Non-Food Sources:

Inositol comes in a tablet and in a powdered form. The powdered form is very expensive because reports indicate Inositol is used to cut Cocaine.

Side Effects and Toxicity:

There are no known adverse effects or toxicity for Inositol.

PABA (Para-aminobenzoic Acid)

Recommended Daily Allowance:

300 - 400 mg

Type: Water Soluble Vitamin

Some Food Sources for PABA:

Bran, Brewer's yeast, Eggs, Liver, Milk, Molasses, Organ meats, Muscle meats, Rice, Yeast, Wheat germ

Side Effects and Toxicity:

Some common side effects of PABA are skin rash and loss of appetite.

Some adverse effects and toxicity of PABA are realized when taking doses greater than 12 gm / day and are leukopenia, fever, liver disease, malaise, rare cases of fatal idiosyncratic reactions have been reported and rash.

PABA may interfere with Sulfonamides and may increase the effect of Corticosteroids.

Calcium

Recommended Daily Allowance

1,000 mg
1,500 mg for males over age 65
1,200 - 1,500 mg during pregnancy
1,500 mg for females post-menopausal, without estrogen

Type: Major Mineral

Some Food Sources for Calcium:

Almonds, Sardines, Salmon, Blackstrap Molasses, Sesame seeds, Buttermilk, Cheddar cheese, Clove of garlic, Shrimp, Milk, Trout, Goat's milk, Yogurt

Side Effects and Toxicity:

Calcium and magnesium compete for GI absorption and excessive thyroid hormone may cause excessive excretion of calcium from bone loss. High calcium (2,000 mg / day) can decrease iron and manganese absorption. High zinc (150 mg / day) leads to decrease in calcium absorption. If no magnesium is used, calcium may exacerbate dioxin toxicity. An increase in sodium intake can lead to an increase in calcium in the urine and increased phosphorus leads

305

to a decrease in active vitamin D and therefore a decrease in calcium. Corticosteroids cause calcium depletion and Tetracycline inhibit calcium absorption.

Phosphorus

Recommended Daily Allowance:

800 mg
1,200 mg during pregnancy

Type: Major Mineral

Some Food Sources for Phosphorus:

Dairy products, Fish, Beef, Poultry, Eggs, Legumes, Grains

Side Effects and Toxicity:

Relative deficiency of calcium which could lead to Hypocalcemia.

Magnesium

Recommended Daily Allowance:

350 mg for males
300 mg for females
320 mg during pregnancy
355 mg for females lactating 0-6 months
340 mg for females lactating 6 months +

Type: Major Mineral

Some Food Sources for Magnesium:

Almonds, Peas, Barley, Pecans, Brazil nuts, Pumpkin seeds, Brown rice, Rye, Buckwheat, Sesame seeds, Carrots, Sunflower seeds, Cashews, Walnuts, Corn, Wheat bran, Filberts, Wheat germ, Mineral water

Side Effects and Toxicity:

Large doses of Magnesium may cause diarrhea. If taken by injection, it may cause a persistent lump at the injection site and Magnesium may cause hypertension. Magnesium may also reduce the effectiveness of lithium in treating patients with bipolar disorder.

Sodium

Recommended Daily Allowance:

No more than 2,400 to 3,000 mg
Minimum 500 mg

Type: Major Mineral

Some Food Sources for Sodium:

Table salt, Soy sauce, Pickled foods, Canned foods, Many processed foods

Side Effects and Toxicity:

Excesses in Sodium may cause hypertension.

Chloride

307

Recommended Daily Allowance:

750 mg

Type: Major Mineral

Some Food Sources for Chloride:
(Usually consumed as Sodium Chloride)

Table salt, Soy sauce

Side Effects and Toxicity:

Although rare, side effects include possible vomiting and a disturbed acid-base.

Potassium

Recommended Daily Allowance:

2,000 mg

Type: Major Mineral

Some Food Sources for Potassium:

Fruit, Vegetables, Dairy Products, Grains, Beef

Side Effects and Toxicity:

Some common side effects of Potassium are muscular weakness and possible vomiting.

Sulfur

Recommended Daily Allowance:

No RDA has been established for Sulfur, as this mineral is a component of Supplements such as Biotin, Thiamin, insulin, some amino acids

Type: Major Mineral

Some Food Sources for Sulfur:

All protein-containing foods

Side Effects and Toxicity:

At this time, side effects and toxicity are unknown as they only occur with excess of certain amino acids.

Iodine

Recommended Daily Allowance:

150 mg
175 mg during pregnancy
200 mg during lactation

Type: Trace Mineral

Some Food Sources for Iodine:

Iodized salt, Bread, Seafood

Side Effects and Toxicity:

Depressed thyroid activity.

Iron

Recommended Daily Allowance:

10 mg for adult males
15 mg for females ages 11 - 50
10 mg for female's ages 50+
30 mg during pregnancy
15 mg during lactation

Type: Trace Mineral

Some Food Sources for Iron:

Beef, Fish, Poultry, Shellfish, Eggs, Legumes, Dried
fruits, Fortified cereals

Side Effects and Toxicity:

Infections, liver damage, possible increased cancer
and heart disease risk.

Zinc

Recommended Daily Allowance:

15 mg males
12 mg for females
15 mg pregnant and lactation

Type: Trace Mineral

Some Food Sources for Zinc:

Oysters, Corn meal, Meats, Black-eyed peas, Egg
yolk, Green peas, Seafood, Garbanzo beans, Soy
meal, Lentil, Wheat bran, Lima beans, Buckwheat,

Pumpkin seeds, Millet rice bran, Peanuts, Whole wheat flour, Spinach, Oatmeal, Onions, Brown rice, Corn meal

Side Effects and Toxicity:

Some adverse effects of Zinc are anemia, nausea, skin rashes, gastritis, and depression and alcohol intolerance.

When taking Zinc without Copper supplementation, you may experience cardiac arrhythmia, impaired immunity. Do not supplement zinc without supplementing copper (ratio of 8:1)

Copper

Recommended Daily Allowance

1.5 - 3 mg

Type: Trace mineral

Some Food Sources for Copper

Brazil nuts, Cashews, Dried fruits, Drinking water, Mushrooms, Organ meats, Sesame seeds, Shellfish, Walnuts, Yeast

Side Effects and Toxicity:

Some adverse side effects from Copper are chronic large doses of copper may cause cirrhosis of the liver, depression, diarrhea in children, insomnia, joint pain, muscle pain, nausea or vomiting and poor memory.

Toxicity is rarely seen except in patients with Wilson's disease or from contaminated water.

Fluoride

Estimated Safe and Adequate Daily Dietary Intakes:

3.8 mg males
3.1 mg females

Type: Trace Mineral

Some Food Sources for Fluoride:

Drinking water (if fluoridated), Tea, Seafood

Side Effects and Toxicity:

Fluorosis, known as discolored teeth

Selenium

Recommended Daily Allowance:

70 mg for males
55 mg for females
65 mg during pregnancy
76 mg during lactation

Type: Trace Mineral

Some food sources for Selenium:

Brewer's yeast, Fish, Organ meats, Whole grains

Side Effects and Toxicity:

When taking Selenium, large doses may cause hair loss, nail loss, nausea, vomiting, fatigue, diarrhea, irritability, dermatological lesions, digestive disorders and a garlic odor. It is suggested that you do not take Selenium on an empty stomach.

Chromium

Estimated Safe and Adequate Daily Dietary Intake:

50 - 200 mg

Type: Trace Mineral

Some Food Sources for Chromium:

Brewer's yeast, Fruits, Vegetables, Vegetable oils, Whole grains, Sunflower seeds, Pumpkin seeds

Side Effects and Toxicity:

Limited primarily to occupational exposure (non-dietary) in Hexavalent Chromium.

Molybdenum

Estimated Safe and Adequate Dietary Intakes:

75 - 250 mg

Type: Trace Mineral

Some Food Sources for Molybdenum:

Cereals, Legumes, Organ meat, Leafy vegetables

Side Effects and Toxicity:

Enzyme inhibition and gout.

Manganese

Estimated Safe and Adequate Dietary Intakes:

2 - 5 mg

Type: Trace Mineral

Some Food Sources for Manganese:

Fruits, Vegetables, Pecans, Peanuts, Fruit juice, Oatmeal, Rice

Side Effects and Toxicity:

Although rare, Nervous system disorders and schizophrenia sometimes occurs. Most over exposure to Manganese are occupational exposures.

Cobalt

Recommended Daily Allowance:

No RDA has been established for Cobalt.

Type: Trace Mineral

Some Food Sources for Cobalt:

Meat, Dairy products, Green leafy vegetables

Side Effects and Toxicity:

There are no known side effects or toxicity associated with Cobalt.

Histidine

Recommended Daily Allowance:

8 - 10 mg

Type: Essential Amino Acid

Some Food Sources for Histidine:

Pork, Poultry, Rice, Wheat, Cheese

Side Effects and Toxicity:

Possible anxiety disorders, stress.

Isoleucine

Recommended Daily Allowance:

10 mg

Type: Essential Amino Acid, Branched Chain
Amino Acid

Some Food Sources for Isoleucine:

Eggs, Fish, Lentils, Poultry, Beef, Sunflower seeds, Pumpkin seeds, Soy, Wheat, Almonds, Dairy products

Some Side Effects and Toxicity:

Elevated urination.

Leucine

Recommended Daily Allowance

14 mg

Type: Essential Amino Acid, Branched Chain
Amino Acid

Some Food Sources for Leucine:

Eggs, Fish, Lentils, Poultry, Beef, Sunflower seeds,
Pumpkin seeds, Soy, Wheat, Almonds, Dairy
products, Beans, Brown rice

Side Effect and Toxicity:

Hypoglycemia, possible Pellagra.

Lysine

Recommended Daily Allowance:

12 mg

Type: Essential Amino Acid

Some Food Sources for Lysine:

Fish, Eggs, Dairy products, Lima beans, Beef, Soy,
Yeast, Potatoes

Side Effects and Toxicity:

There are no known side effects or toxicity associated with Lysine.

Methionine

Recommended Daily Allowance:

13 mg

Type: Essential Amino Acid

Some Food Sources for Methionine:

Fish, Eggs, Dairy products, Beans, Beef, Garlic, Onion, Lentils, Soybeans

Side Effects and Toxicity:

There are no known side effects or toxicity associated with Methionine.

Phenylalanine

Recommended Daily Allowance:

14 mg

Type: Essential Amino Acid

Some Food Sources for Phenylalanine:

Dairy products, Almonds, Avocados, Lima beans, Peanuts, Sunflower seeds, Pumpkin seeds

Side Effect and Toxicity:

Although rare, decreased / increased blood pressure, headaches.

Threonine

Recommended Daily Allowance:

7 mg

Type: Essential Amino Acid

Some Food Sources for Threonine:

Beans, Beef, Dairy products, Eggs, Nuts, Poultry, Beans, Sunflower seeds, Pumpkin seeds

Side Effects and Toxicity:

There are no known side effects or toxicity associated with Threonine.

Tryptophan

Recommended Daily Allowance

3.5 mg

Tryptophan supplementation has been determined unsafe and is illegal in the United States.

Type: Essential Amino Acid

Some Food Sources for Tryptophan:

Barley, Beef, Brown rice, Dairy products, Fish,
Peanuts, Poultry, Soybeans

Side Effects and Toxicity:

There are no know sided effects or toxicity
associated with Tryptophan, however, Eosinophilia-
myalgia syndrome (potentially fatal) resulted from a
contaminated batch of supplemental Tryptophan:
resulting in a ban from the FDA.

Valine

Recommended Daily Allowance:

10 mg

Type: Essential Amino Acid, Branched Chain
        Amino Acid

Some Food Sources for Valine:

Beef, Dairy products, Eggs, Grain, Mushrooms,
Nuts, Poultry, Soy

Side Effects and Toxicity:

Possible hallucinations

Alanine

Recommended Daily Allowance:

No RDA has been established for Alanine.

Type: Non-Essential Amino Acid
319

Some Food Sources for Alanine:

Avocado, Beef, Dairy products, Poultry, Wheat

Side Effects and Toxicity:

There are no known side effects or toxicity associated with Alanine.

Arginine

Recommended Daily Allowance:

No RDA has been established for Arginine.

Type: Non-Essential Amino Acid

Some Food Sources for Arginine:

Brown rice, Carob, Chocolate, Peanuts, Popcorn, Pumpkin seeds, Raisins, Soy, Sunflower seeds, Whole wheat

Side Effects and Toxicity:

Although rare, weakness, diarrhea, nausea, may increase the activity of some viruses.

Asparagine

Recommended Daily Allowance:

No RDA has been established for Asparagine.

Type: Non-Essential Amino Acid

Some Food Sources for Asparagine:

Beef, Dairy products, Eggs, Poultry

Side Effects and Toxicity:

There are no known side effects or toxicity associated with Asparagine.

Aspartic acid

Recommended Daily Allowance:

No RDA has been established for Aspartic acid.

Type: Non-Essential Amino Acid

Some Food Sources for Aspartic acid:

Beef, Dairy products, Poultry, Sprouting seeds

Side Effects and Toxicity:

There are no side effects or toxicity associated with Aspartic acid.

Cysteine

Recommended Daily Allowance:

No RDA has been established for Cysteine.

Type: Non-Essential Amino Acid

Some Food Sources for Cysteine:

Brussel sprouts, Broccoli, Eggs, Garlic, Onions, Poultry, Red peppers, Wheat

Side Effects and Toxicity:

There are no known side effects or toxicity associated with Cysteine.

Glutamic acid

Recommended Daily Allowance:

No RDA has been established for Glutamic acid.

Type: Non-Essential Amino Acid

Some Food Sources for Glutamic acid:

Found abundantly in most foods.

Side Effects and Toxicity:

Possible headaches, neurological problems.

Glycine

Recommended Daily Allowance:

No RDA has been established for Glycine.

Type: Non-Essential Amino Acid

Glycine is produced in the body.

Side Effects and Toxicity:

322

There are no known side effects or toxicity associated with Glycine.

Proline

Recommended Daily Allowance:

No RDA has been established for Proline.

Type: Non-Essential Amino Acid

Some Food Sources for Proline:

Beef, Dairy products, Eggs, Poultry, Wheat

Side Effects and Toxicity:

There are no known side effects or toxicity associated with Proline.

Serine

Recommended Daily Allowance:

No RDA has been established for Serine.

Type: Non-Essential Amino Acid

Some Food Sources for Serine:

Beef, Dairy products, Peanuts, Poultry, Soy, Wheat gluten

Side Effects and Toxicity:

There are no known side effects or toxicity associated with Serine.

Tyrosine

Recommended Daily Allowance:

No RDA has been established for Tyrosine.

Type: Non-Essential Amino Acid

Some Food Sources for Tyrosine:

Almonds, Avocados, Bananas, Beef, Dairy products, Eggs, Fish, Lima beans, Pumpkin seeds, Sesame seeds, Soy

Side Effects and Toxicity:

There are no known side effects or toxicity associated with Tyrosine.

Glutamine

Recommended Daily Allowance:

No RDA has been established for Glutamine.

Type: Non-Essential Amino Acid

Some Food Sources for Glutamine:

Raw parsley, Spinach   (Found abundantly in many foods)

Side Effects and Toxicity

Possible decrease of growth hormone and may interfere with acid-base balance in the body.

Althea officinalis (Marshmallow)

Recommended Daily Allowance

RDA has not been established for Althea officinlis.

Some of the therapeutic actions of Althea officinalis is that it acts as an:

Anti-inflammatory
Antispasmodic
Demulcent
Stimulates IL-1
Stimulates T and B cell activity
Vulnerary
Relieves pain from inflamed mucosal tissues
Gastritis
Pharyngitis
Vaginitis
Relieves external pain for:
    All inflammatory skin disorders
    Burns
    Ulcers
    Wounds

Some of the side effects of Althea officinalis is that anti-inflammatory activity escalates the effects of topical steroids and any oral drugs or herbs taken with marshmallow may have delayed absorption due to the mucilage content.

There is no known toxicity associated with Althea officinalis.

Curcuma longa (Tumeric)

Recommended Daily Allowance:

RDA has not been established for Curcuma longa.

Some of the therapeutic actions of Curcuma longa is that is acts as an:

Analgesic
Anticoagulant
Antifertility action
Anti-inflammatory
Antimicrobial
Antineoplastic
Antioxidant
Antiplatelet-aggregator
Carminative
Cholagogue
Emmenagogue
Hepatoprotective
Hypotensive
Increases glutathione content in liver
Increases rate-limiting step of cholesterol conversion into bile acids
Inhibits platelet aggregation
Inhibits lymphocytic activity
Lowers LDL cholesterol and raises HDL cholesterol
Stabilizes lysosomal membranes
Stimulates digestive enzymes
Topical antibacterial and antifungal
Tumor-preventing activity

There is no known side effects or toxicity associated with Curcuma longa

Echinacea angustifolia (Purple cone flower)

Recommended Daily Allowance:

RDA has not been established for Echinacea angusstifolia.

Some of the therapeutic actions of Althea officinalis is that is acts as an:

Alterative
Antibacterial
Antifungal
Anti-inflammatory
Antiviral - both RNA and DNA viruses
Activates macrophages to cytotoxicity
    against tumor cells and micro-organisms,
    producing tumor necrosis factor (TNF),
    interleukin-1, interleukin-6, interferon-2 and
    slight increase in T-lymphocyte proliferation
Decreases inflammatory allergic reactions to mild
food allergies
    Immune stimulating:
    Enhances antibody binding
    Enhances antibody dependent cytotoxicity
    Enhances phagocytosis
    Improves carbon clearance
    Interferon activation
    Inhibits hyaluronidase
    Root oil has inhibited leukemia cells in vitro and
    in vivo
  Slight stimulation of the adrenal cortex

327

There are no known adverse effects or toxicity associated with Echinacea angustifolia

Essential Fatty Acids (EFAs)

Essential Fatty Acids come in two forms

Supplement Form 1 (Omega 3)

Alpha-linolenic (ALA) - flaxseed, soy, linseed oil, chloroplasts

Eicosapentanoic acid (EPA) - salmon, herring, sardine, mackerel, etc.

Physiologic Therapeutics (Omega 3 - EPA 3 - 10 gm in divided doses)

Alters eicosanoid production
Decreases blood cholesterol
Decrease platelet aggregation
Decreases triglycerides
Enhances lymph function
Increases exercise tolerance
Increases HDL
Precursor for 3 prostaglandins (PGE 3)
Suppresses division in cancer cell lines

Supplement Form 2 (Omega 6)

Linoleic - vegetable, nut, and seed oils and evening primrose oil

Gamma-linolenic (GLA) - breast milk, evening primrose, black currant, and borage oils

Physiologic Therapeutics (Omega 6 EPO 2 - 4 gm)

Decreases blood cholesterol
Decreases platelet aggregation
GLA decreases growth of malignant cell lines in
    vitro
PGE 1 decreases kidney damage in mice
PGE 1 needed for T-lymphocyte function
Precursor for 1 prostaglandins (PGE 1)

These Vitamins require vitamin E and possibly other
antioxidants when ingesting large doses

Keep unsaturated oils in refrigerator

Taking large doses of Omega 3 or Omega 6 may cause
peroxidation damage if taken without antioxidant
supplementation

Fructooliogosaccharides (FOS)

FOS, short-chain polysaccharides, is soluble fiber
from edible plants.   Certain lactic acid producing
probiotic microflora, Lactobacilli and Bifidobacteria,
utilize FOS as food.

Recommended Daily Allowance

2,000 - 3,000 mg

Some Plants / Food which contain FOS:

Asparagus, Garlic, Jerusalem artichokes, Onions

Some of the therapeutic actions of FOS:

Enhances elimination of toxic substances
Feeds the friendly gut bacteria
Improves liver function
Increases production of butyrate, a beneficial short-chain fatty acid
Increases Lactobacilli and Bifidobacteria
Reduces cholesterol
Reduces detrimental bacteria
Reduces hypertension

Side Effects and Toxicity:

There are no known adverse effects or toxicity associated with FOS.

Geranium maculatum (Wild geranium, Cranesbill)

Recommended Daily Allowance:

RDA has not been established for Geranium maculatum.

Some of the therapeutic actions of Geranium maculatum are that it helps:

Astringent
Atonic tissues with discharges due to over-relaxation
Diarrhea
Passive hemorrhages
Styptic
Ulceration or inflammation of the mucous membranes and digestive tract
Geranium maculatum and Hydrastis together tend to stop intestinal bleeding and suppuration

Chronic or sub acute bowel disorders - dries long-standing thick secretions, promotes solid stool formation

Side Effects and Toxicity:

There are no known adverse effects or toxicity associated with Geranium maculatum.

DO NOT TAKE GERANUM MACULATUM IF YOU ARE EXPERIENCING HEAVY BLEEDING. SEE YOUR DOCTOR

Glycyrrhiza glabra (Licorice)

Recommended Daily Allowance:

RDA has not been established for Glycyrrhiza glabra.

Some of the therapeutic actions of Glycyrrhiza glabra:

Adrenal-modulator
Anti-allergic
Antibacterial
Antioxidant
Antiviral
Decreases inflammation by enhancing movement of
    leukocytes towards inflamed areas
Immune stimulating
Laxative
Liver tonic and protectant
Spasmolytic
Steroidal - estrogenic
Stimulates natural killer cell activity

Some of the Drug / Nutrient interactions that you should be aware of:

Corticoid treatment - Glycyrrhizin glabra interferes with 5 beta-reductase breakdown of corticosteroids, thus prolonging its biological half-life
Potentiates hypokalemia and sodium retention when used with insulin
Potentiates potassium loss when used with diuretics like thiazides
Potentiates potassium loss when used with stimulant laxatives
Potentiates the activity of anthraquinone drugs or herbs containing anthraquinones
Potentiates the toxicity of cardiac glycosides like digitalis due to potassium loss in the urine
Reduces ulcer formation caused by aspirin intake

Chronic use of Glycyrhrza glabra may mimic aldosteronism by increasing sodium resorption and potassium excretion by the kidney. Some of the symptoms you may experience are edema, headache, hypertension, hypokalemia and vertigo.

Humulus lupulus (Hops)

Recommended Daily Allowance:

RDA has not been established Humulus lupulus.

Some of the therapeutic actions of Humulus lupulus:

Relaxes smooth muscles, especially in the digestive tract; Anaphrodisiac for men due to the estrogenic substances; Diuretic due to asparagin; Antibacterial due to humulone and lupulone; Antispasmodic effect on uteri in animal studies; Anti inflammatory, especially in the areas of the digestive tract; Sedative, promotes sleep; Astringent

When taking Humulus lupulus, you may experience a marked depression due to the sedative effect. Contact with the pollen from the strobiles may cause dermatitis

Hydrastis canadensis (Goldenseal)

Recommended Daily Allowance:

RDA has not been established for Hydrastis canadensis.

Some of the therapeutic actions of Hydrastis canadensis:

Adrenolytic
Antimicrobia against:
    Amebiasis, bacteria, cholera, giardia, protozoa,
        visceral and cutaneous leishmaniasis, yeast
Astringent
Enhances splenic blood flow
Bitter tonic
Immune support
Increases macrophage activity
Laxative in small doses
Stimulates the normal action of the liver and gall bladder
Styptic
Triples bile secretion for 1.5 hours
In vitro was a potent macrophage activator for inducing cytostatic activity against tumor cells

Side Effects and Toxicity:

Some of the adverse effects that Hydrastis canadensis may have are hypoglycemia and it may deplete B vitamins.

Some of the toxicity of Hydrastis canadensis is that it may cause catarrhal inflammation of the mucous linings of the hepatic ducts and gall bladder, causing an icteric hue to skin; and continued large doses may cause ulceration of mucous membranes with extreme dryness and fissure formation.

Lactobacillus Acidophilus and Bifidus (Probiotics)

Recommended Daily Allowance:

Based on the number of live bacteria

1 - 10 billion viable Acidophilus or Bifidus

Some of the therapeutic actions of Acidophilus and Bifidus:

Reduces production of procarcinogens
Inhibits the growth of:
 Clostridium perfringens
 Bacillus subtilis
 Candida ablicans
 Escherichia coli
 Bacillus cereus
 Klebsiella pneumoniae
 Proteus vulgaris
 L. bulgaricus
 L. fermenti

L. lactis
L. plantarum
L. helveticus
L. leichmannii
    Helps maintain optimum pH
    Reduces putrefaction
    Reduces endotoxemia

Side Effects and Toxicity:

Antibiotics and alcohol negatively affect Acidophilus and Bifidus.

There are no adverse affects or toxicity associated with Acidophilus or Bifidus.

Acidophilus and Bifidus are two of the most important strains of the Lactobacilli family of microflora which inhibit the gastrointestinal tract. These "good" bacteria are involved with immune system function, carcinogenesis, metabolism of cholesterol, aging, and nutritional status. The term probiotics is used to describe the health-promoting effects of friendly bacteria in the gut.

Mentha piperita (Peppermint)

Recommended Daily Allowance:

RDA has not been established for Mentha piperita.

Some of the therapeutic actions of Mentha piperita are:

    Analgesic, topical
    Anti-inflammatory
    Antinuclear properties

335

Block calcium influx into muscle cells causing inhibition of isolated contractions
Calms and strengthens nerves
Calms an upset stomach
Decreases flaccidity in the GI tract
Digestive aid
Dissolves gallstones
Eliminates heartburn
Improves solubility of bile
Increases bile acid and lecithin levels in the gallbladder
Inhibits and kills micro-organisms:
Candida albicans, herpes simplex, influenza A viruses, mumps virus, Pseudomonas acruginosa, Streptococcus pyogenes, Staphylococcus aureus
Inhibits constipation
Inhibits diarrhea
Inhibits hypercontractility of intestinal smooth muscle
Mild anaesthetic to stomach wall
Normalizes gastrointestinal activity
Prevents congestion of blood to the brain
Reduces bile cholesterol levels
Stimulates circulation
Stimulates contractile activity and bile secretion in the gallbladder

Side Effects and Toxicity:

Mentha piperita may cause hypersensitivity and result in bradycardia, heartburn, muscle tremor and skin rash.

Quercetin

Recommended Daily Allowance:

400 mg (20 minutes before meals)

Some Plants / Food Which Contain Quercetin:

Apple	Hydrangea
Asparagus	Kale
Bearberry	Pale catechu
Bell peppers	Passion flower
Black catechu	Pear
Boneset	Podophyllum
Brussel Sprouts	Onion
Dill	Squill
Elder flowers	Tarragon
Eucalyptus	Tea
Euphorbia	Witch-hazel
Fenugreek	

Side Effects and Toxicity:

There are no known adverse effects or toxicity associated with Quercetin.

Quercetin is the glycone of quercitrin, rutin and other flavonoids. Glycosides are compounds that yield one or more sugars among the products of hydrolysis. The non-sugar component is known as the aglycone, and the sugar component is called glycogen. The flavonoid glycosides and their aglycones are generally termed flavonoids. Rutin, quercitrin, and the citrus bioflavonoids, including hesperidin, hesperetin, diosmin, and naringen, are among the best known flavonoid constituents.

Ulmus fulva (Slippery elm, American elm)

337

Recommended Daily Allowance:

RDA has not been established for Ulmus fulva.

Some of the therapeutic actions of Ulmus fulva are:

Demulcent - used to soothe irritated mucosal tissues
Nutritive
Vulnerary

Side Effects and Toxicity:

There are no known adverse effects or toxicity
associated with Ulmus fulva.

Chapter 16

Herbs and Herbalism

Oriental Medicine

According to the theories of Oriental medicine, Crohn's disease may be caused by constitutional deficiencies, invasion of the exterior pathogenic factors, or unbalanced diet. Constitutional deficiencies usually refer to spleen and kidney deficiencies. Invasion of exterior pathogenic factors refers to damp heat in the large intestine. Lastly, unbalanced diet high in raw or cold injures the spleen and stomach and obstructs their functions in transforming and transporting food and nutrients.

Differential Diagnosis

Crohn's disease can be divided into four general categories: damp heat; spleen deficiency, spleen and kidney deficiencies, and Qi and blood stagnation.

Invasion of damp heat in the large intestine is characterized by an acute and sudden onset of gastrointestinal symptoms. Damp heat in the large intestine is illustrated by diarrhea, presence of mucous and blood in the stool, foul-smelling stools, yellow urine, and abdominal fullness and pain. As heat travels upwards, patients may feel irritable, thirsty, and have a preference to drink cold water. The tongue is dark red with a yellow, greasy coat; the pulse is wiry, slippery or rapid.

Spleen deficiency may be due to constitutional deficiency or secondary due to excessive intake of cold and raw food. Patients with chronic Crohn's disease usually have spleen deficiency, which is characterized by a compromised ability of the spleen to transform and transport food. Clinically, the patient will show symptoms such as frequent and severe diarrhea, watery stool with undigested food, dull abdominal pain, poor appetite, poor digestion, and gastric discomfort after food intake. Sallow facial appearance, fatigue and lethargy are due to chronic malabsorption and malnutrition. The tongue is pale with a white coat; the pulse is soft and weak.

Spleen and kidney deficiencies may be due to constitutional deficiency or secondary due to chronic nature of the illness. One diagnostic key of spleen and kidney deficiency is early morning diarrhea around 5:00 am. In addition, patients may have abdominal pain that increases with cold but decreases with defecation. Patients may also have intolerance to cold and cold extremities. The tongue is pale with a white coat; the pulse is thready and weak.

Lastly, *qi* and blood stagnation resembles an acute phase of Crohn's disease in which the patient has severe abdominal pain and fullness with a palpable mass in the right lower quadrant. This condition mimics acute appendicitis. It is essential to make a correct differential diagnosis prior to treatment. In addition, patients may experience diarrhea, lack of appetite, muscle wasting and lethargy. The tongue is dark purple with petechia; the pulse is thready and knotted.

Herbal Treatment

340

Damp heat in the Xia Jiao, or lower burner, causes an acute and sudden onset of gastrointestinal symptoms and signs such as diarrhea, presence of mucous and blood in the stool, foul-smelling stools, yellow urine, abdominal fullness and pain, extreme urgency to defecate, tenesmus, burning sensation of the anus after passing stools, irritability, thirst, preference to drink cold water, dark red tongue, yellow, greasy tongue coat, wiry, slippery, or rapid pulse.

Herbal Formula

Peony combination (*shao yao tang*). This formula eliminates damp heat and toxin from the *xia jiao* and is commonly used to treat inflammation of the intestines.

Modifications

Excessive heat and toxin: add pulsatilla (*bai tou weng*) and dandelion (*pu gong ying*)

Excessive damp: add coix (*yi yi ren*) and poria (*fu ling*)

Abdominal fullness and swelling: add scirpus (*sang leng*) and zedoaria (*e zhu*)

Spleen & Kidney Deficiency

A spleen deficiency will cause frequent and severe diarrhea, watery stool with undigested food, dull abdominal pain, poor appetite, poor digestion, gastric discomfort after food intake, sallow facial appearance, fatigue, lethargy, pale tongue with white tongue coat, soft and weak pulse.

341

Herbal Formula

Ginseng & atractylodes formula (*shen ling bai zhu san*). This formula tonifies qi and strengthens the spleen and stomach. It may be used for chronic diarrhea due to enteritis.

Crohn's formula. This formula is called a *yan fan* (an experienced formula). It is not a classic herbal formula, but one designed with years of clinical experience specifically for treating chronic Crohn's disease with deficiencies of *qi*, blood, spleen and kidney. Ingredients and dosage is as follows: salvia (*dan shen*), 15g; red peony (*chi shao*), 12g; white peony (*bai shao*), 12g; white atractylodes (*bai zhu*), 9g; angelica sinensis (*dang gui*), 12g; carthamus (*hong hua*), 9g; cinidium (*chuan xiong*), 9g; codonopsis (*dang shen*), 12g; aurantium fruit (*zhi ke*), 9g; saussurea (*mu xiang*), 9g; citrus peel (*chen pi*), 9g; pinellia (*ban xia*), 9g; and licorice (*gan cao*), 4g.

Modifications

If you have a poor appetite, add crataegus (*sha zha*), massa medicata fermenta (*shen qu*) and barley sprouts (*mai ya*).

If you are experiencing watery diarrhea due to spleen deficiency with interior cold then add decoction to regulate the spleen and stomach (*li zhong wan*) plus prepared aconite (*fu zi*) and cinnamon bark (*rou gui*).

Spleen and Kidney Deficiencies

You are probably experiencing spleen and kidney deficiencies if you have early morning diarrhea at around 5:00 am, abdominal pain which increases with cold but decreases with defecation, aversion to cold/cold extremities, pale tongue with white tongue coat, thready and weak pulse.

Herbal Formula

Pills of four miraculous drugs (*si shen wan*). This is an effective herbal formula to treat diarrhea due to spleen and kidney deficiencies. Codonopsis and white atractylodes are added to increase its overall effect to tonify *qi* and strengthen the spleen.

Modifications

If you have severe diarrhea, add terminalia (*he zi*), rubrum halloysitum (*chi shi zi*) and limonitum (*yu liang shi*).

If you are experiencing cold extremities, add prepared aconite and cinnamon bark.

Qi Deficiency and Blood Stagnation

If you have a Qi deficiency or blood stagnation, you will experience severe abdominal pain and fullness with a palpable mass in the right lower quadrant, diarrhea, lack of appetite, muscle wasting, lethargy, dark purple tongue with petechia, and a thready and knotted pulse.

Herbal Formula

Tangkuei & corydalis combination (*ge xia zhu yu tang*). This formula is commonly used to relieve pain in the abdominal region due to *qi* and blood stagnation.

Modifications

343

If you have diarrhea, add crataegus (*shan zha*), terminalia and dioscorea (*shan yao*). For a *Qi* deficiency: add codonopsis and white atractylodes.

The information for this Chapter on Herbs and Herbalism was used with the gracious permission of Dr. John K. Chen. For further information on Herbs and Herbalism, you may contact Mr. Chen at JohnChen@lotusherbs.com.

Author's note: Parts of Dr. Chen's original article appeared in the November 2000 issue of *Acupuncture Today.*

Chapter 17

Organizations

The following organizations are available to further assist you in dealing with your Crohn's, its side effects and other related diseases. There are many more organizations that are available; this is just a small sampling of what is actually out there. Check your local telephone directory, public library or the Internet for other organizations and sites. Some information for this book was acquired from several of the organizations listed below.

Crohn's & Colitis Foundation of America, Inc.
386 Park Avenue South, 17th Floor
New York, NY 10016
Phone: (800) 932-2423
Fax: (212) 779-4098

Pediatric Crohn's & Colitis Association, Inc.
P. O. Box 188
Newton, Massachusetts 02468
Phone: (617) 489-5854

Crohn's and Colitis Foundation of Canada
21 St. Clair Avenue East, Suite 301
Toronto, Ontario
M4T 1L9 Canada
Phone: (416) 920-5035

Phone: (800) 387-1479

National Institute of Diabetes and Digestive and Kidney Disorders
31 Center Dr.
Bethesda, MD 20892
Phone: (301) 496-3583
Fax: (301) 496-7422

Reach Out for Youth with Ileitis and Colitis, Inc.
15 Chemung Place
Jericho, NY 11753
Phone: (516) 822-8010

United Ostomy Association, Inc.
19772 MacArthur Blvd., #200
Irvine, CA 92612-2405
Phone: (800) 826-0826
Phone: (949) 660-8624
Fax: (949) 660-9262

National Digestive Diseases Information Clearinghouse
2 Information Way
Bethesda, MD 20892-3570

American Liver Foundation
75 Maiden Ln.
Suite 603
New York, NY 10038
Phone: (800) 465-4837

American College of Gastroenterology (ACG)
4900 B South, 31st St.
Arlington, VA 22206
Phone: (703) 820-7400

Fax: (703) 931-4520

American Auto-Immune Related Diseases Association (AARDA)
22100 Gratiot Ave.
East Detroit, MI 48021
Phone: (810) 776-3900

National Institutes of Health
National Heart Lung Blood Institute (NHLBI)
P.O. Box 30105
Bethesda, MD 20824-0105
Phone: (301) 592-8573
Fax: (301) 592-8563

National Diabetes Information Clearinghouse
1 Information Way
Bethesda, MD 20892-3560
Phone: (301) 654-3327

Arthritis Foundation
1330 West Peachtree Street
Atlanta, GA 30309
Phone: (404) 872-7100
Phone: (800) 283-7800

Spondylitis Association of America
14827 Ventura Blvd., #222
Sherman Oaks, CA 91403
Phone: (800) 777-8189
Phone: (818) 981-1616

The North American Spine Society
22 Calendar Court, 2nd Floor
LaGrange, IL 60525
Phone: (877 Spine-Dr

Phone: (847) 698-1630.
American College of Rheumatology
1800 Century Place, Suite 250
Atlanta, GA 30345
Phone: (404) 633-3777
Fax: (404) 633-1870

Molo-Cure Research, Inc.
4631 NW 31st Ave., #247
Fort Lauderdale, FL 33309
Phone: (888) 858-4300
Phone: (954) 941-5521
Fax: (954) 941-5562

MedicineNet.com
903 Calle Amanecer, Suite 300
San Clemente, CA 92673
Phone: (949) 940-6500
Fax: (949) 940-1094

Centocor, Inc. Medical Affairs
Medical Information Department
200 Great Valley Parkway
Malvern, PA 19355
Phone (800) 457-6399

American Academy of Environmental Medicine
4510 W. 89th St., Suite 110
Prairie Village, Kansas, 66207-2282
Phone: (913) 642-6062

US Food and Drug Administration,
5600 Fishers Lane
Rockville, MD 20857-0001
Phone: (888) INFO-FDA

US Department of Health and Human Services
200 Independence Ave. SW
Washington, DC 20201
Phone: (877) 696-6776

Centers for Disease Control and Prevention
1600 Clifton Road
Atlanta, GA 30333
Phone: (404) 639-3311

The National Pancreas Foundation
P.O. Box 935
Wexford, PA 15090-0935

US Department of Agriculture
Center for Nutrition Policy and Promotion
1120 20th St., NW
Suite 200, North Lobby
Washington, DC 20036-3475

International Foundation for Functional
Gastrointestinal Disorders
P.O. Box 170864
Milwaukee, WI 53217
Phone: (888) 964-200

National Association for Colitis and Crohn's Disease
4 Beaumont House
Sutton Road
St Albans, Herts
AL1 5HH.
Phone: +44 (0) 1727 844296

Irritable Bowel Syndrome Network
c/o Centre for Human Nutrition
Northern General Hospital

Sheffield
S5 7AU
Phone 0114 2611531

Digestive Diseases Foundation
3 St Andrew's Place
Regents Park
London NW1 4LB

The Ileostomy and Internal Pouch Support Group
PO Box 123
Scunthorpe
North Lincs
DN15 9YW
Phone: 01724 720150

CANCER BACUP
3 Bath Place
Rivington Street
London EC2A 3JR
Phone: 0800 181199

Continence Advisory Service
The Dene Centre
Castles Farm Road
Newcastle upon Tyne
NE3 1PH
Phone: 0191 213 0050

Crohn's in Childhood Research Association (CICRA)
Parkgate House
356 West Barnes Lane
Motspur Park
Surrey
KT3 6NB
Phone: 020 8949 6209

Fax: 020 8942 2044

British Colostomy Association
15 Station Road
Reading
Berkshire
RG1 1LG
Phone: 0800 328 4257

National Ankylosing Spondilitis Society
PO Box 179
Mayfield
East Sussex
TN20 6ZL
Phone: 01435 873527
Fax: 01435 873027

Austria

Osterreichische Morbus Crohn/Colitis Ulcerosa Vereinigung (OMCCV)
Obere Augartenstrasse 26-28, A-1020
Wien, Austria
Phone: 00 43 1 333 06 33

Israel

The Israel Foundation for Crohn's Disease and Ulcerative Colitis
PO Box 5231 Herzlia,
Israel
Fax: 09 9567628

Belgium

Crohn en Colitis Ulcerosa Vereniging vzw (CCV)
Schalmei 2 B-2970 'S,
Gravenwezel, Belgium
Phone / Fax: 00 32 3 385 2719
Secretary Phone / Fax: 00 32 16 56 83 69

Denmark

Colitis-Crohn-Foreningen (CCF)
Birkegade 11,
2200 Köpenhavn N,
Denmark
Phone: 00 45 31 35 48 82
Fax: 00 45 31 35 47 82

Finland

Crohn ja Colitis ry (CCAFIN)
PO Box 44
02101 Espoo,
Finland
Phone: +358 (0)9 148 5784
Fax: +358 (0)3 241 2561 (Chairman's Office)

France

Association Francois Aupetit (AFA)
Hopital Rothschild,
33 Boulevard de Picpus, 75571,
Paris, Cedex 12,
France
Phone: 00 33 1 40 193 425
Fax: 00 33 1 40 193 436

Germany

**Deutsche Morbus Crohn und Colitis Ulcerosa
Vereinigung, e.V. (DCCV)**
Paracelsusstrasse 15
D-51375 Leverkusen 1,
Germany
Phone: 00 49 214-87608 0
Fax: 00 49 214 87608 88

Hungary

**Magyrarorszagi Crohn-Colitesis Betegek Egyesulete
(MCCBE)**
Igmandi utca 22 Fzst. 1
1112 Budapest
Phone: 00 361 322 8098
Fax: 00 361 457 9494
Secretary Phone / Fax: 00 361 270 0638

Italy

**Associazione per le Malattie Inflammatorie Croniche
dell'Intestino (AMICI)**
c/o Ospendale Nuovo Regina Margherita,
Via Morosini 30,
00153 ROMA
Phone: 06/ 58 33 28 00

**Associazione per le Malattie Inflammatorie Croniche
dell'Intestino (AMICI)**
Via Adolfo Wildt 19/4,
20138 Milano,
Italy
Phone: 00 39 (0)2 28 93 673
Fax: 00 39 (0)2 268 22670

Ireland

The Irish Society for Colitis & Crohn's Disease (ISCC)
Carmichael Centre,
North Brunswick Street, Dublin 7,
Eire
Phone: (353) 1 872 1416
Fax: (353) 1 873 5737

Latvia

Republic Gastroenterological Center
Pilsonu 13, Riga,
Latvia

Lithuania

Vilnius University Children´s Hospital
Center of Pediatry,
Vytauto 15,
2004 Vilnius
Lithuania

Luxembourg

Luxembourg Association Luxembourgeoise de la Maladie de Crohn (ALMC)
PO Box 648, L-2016
Luxembourg
Phone: (352) 50 98 28

The Netherlands

Crohn en Colitis Ulcerosa Vereniging Nederland (CCUVN)

Wilhelminastraat 45, 3621 VG Breukelen,
The Netherlands
Phone: 00 31 346 261001

Norway

Landsforeningen mot Fordoyelessykdommer (LMF)
co FFO Smagruppe-sekretariatet
Postboks 4568 Torshov
0404 Oslo, Norway
Phone: 00 47 88 00 50 21

Portugal

**Associacao Portuguesa de Doenca Inflamatoria do
Intestino (APDI)**
c/o General Chairman
Av. Fernao Magalhaes 476 - Apart 404
3002 Coimbra codex
Fax: 00 351 (0)39 82 93 16

Spain

**Asociacion Nacional de Enfermos de Crohn y Colitis
Ulcerosa (ACCU)**
c/ Hileras 4, 4, 7
28013 Madrid
Phone / Fax: 00 34 9 1542 63 26

Slovakia

Crohn Klub (VUV)
Vyskumny ústav vyzivy,
Limbová 14,
83337 Bratislava

Slovakia

Sweden

Riksförbundet för Mag- och Tarmsjuka (RMT)
Gotlandsgatan 46,
PO Box 20054,
104 60 Stockholm,
Sverige
Tel: +46 (0)8 642 42 00

Switzerland

**Schweizerische Morbus Crohn/Colitis Ulcerosa
Vereinigung (SMCCV)**
Postfach,
5001 Aarau,
Switzerland
Phone / Fax: 00 41(0) 62 824 8707

South Africa

South African Crohn's & Colitis Association
P.O. Box 2638,
Cape Town 800
South Africa
Phone: 021 25-2350

Zimbabwe

Zimbabwe Association for Colitis & Crohn's Disease
2 Montclaire Close
Borrowdale, Harare
Zimbabwe
Phone: Harare 885556

Australia

**The Australian Crohn's and Colitis Association
(ACCA),**
P.O. Box 201, Mooroolbark,
3138, Victoria,
Australia
Phone: (03) 9726 9008

**Australian Crohn's and Colitis Association
(Queensland) (ACCAQ)**
P.O. Box 548, Maleny
Queensland, 4552
Australia
Phone / Fax: (07) 5494 2149

New Zealand

Crohn's & Colitis Support Group Inc.
P.O. Box 52-043,
Kingsland, Auckland,
New Zealand
Phone: +64 9 6367228

This Chapter is included for informational purposes only. The information in these web sites were reviewed and found to be informative, helpful and offered opportunities to learn more about Crohn's disease. Some of them provide a vehicle to contact others who have Crohn's disease by email addresses or chat rooms. I am not personally endorsing of any one web site or any product advertised in any of these web sites.

At the time of the writing of this book, all of these web sites were active. It is possible that listed web sites may be inactive and there may now be more web sites available for you to review.

Keywords

I have found the following Keywords to be very helpful when looking for information on Crohn's disease. There may be many more, but these have given me the greatest results.

> *Crohn's, Crohn's Disease, Irritable Bowel Disease, IBD, Colitis, Ulcerative Colitis, Colon, Digestive System, Gastrointestinal Disorders.*

If there is a particular area that you are looking for, simply type in that word and do a search. Some topics of interest may be fissures, fistula's, sigmoidoscopy, colonoscopy, specific meds, specific procedures and the like.

Search Engines

The most effective and positive search engines I have found are *DogPile, Yahoo, AltaVista, RealNames, DirectHit, Ask Jeeves, Google, Kanoodle, About* and *Overture.*

Web Sites

The following web sites produced the most valuable information about IBD and Crohn's disease. I highly recommend all of these Web Sites to gain more knowledge about Crohn's disease. Some are business sites, some are Government sites and some are personal sites.

www.crohnie.com
crohnie.healingwell.com
www.fda.gov
us.govinfo.about.com
www.medicalmaibox.com
www.askphysicians.com
ibscrohns.about.com
www.ibdpage.com
www.dansac.com
www.healingwell.com
www.angelfire.com
qurlyjoe.bu.edu
www.ccfa.org
www.crohns.net
www.go-symmetry.com
prefdev.ucsd.edu
www.consciouschoice.com

mycrohns.freesavers.com
oldlaces-place.healingwell.com
www.badgut.com
www.e-gastrointestinal.com
www.gentiva.com
ibd.patientcommunity.com
healthlink.mcw.edu
pcca.hypermart.net
www.cdc.gov
www.nacc.org
pages.prodigy.net
www.crohns-support.com
go.to/rachelscrohns
www.living-better.comwww.uel.ac.uk
www.digestivedisorders.org.uk
www.ccfc.ca
www.niddk.nih.gov
www.reachoutforyouth.org
www.uoa.org
www.liverfoudation.org
www.acg.gi.org
www.aarda.org
www.nhlbi.nih.gov
www.arthritis.org
www.spondylitis.org
www.spine.org
www.rheumatology.org
www.molocure.com
www.focusondigestion.com
www.ileostomypouch.demon.co.uk
www.cicra.org
www.oemccv.or.at
www.ccf.dk
www.sci.fi/-ccafin
www.afa.asso.fr
www.dccv.org

www.commune.bologna.it
www.crohn-colitis.nl
www.softlilne.sk
www/vlc.servicom.es
www.accaq.org.au
www.cancerbacup.org.uk
www.pancreasfoundation.com
www.usda.gov

A

Abdominal pain, 38, 39, 42, 48, 50, 52, 55, 56, 64,
67, 68, 70, 71, 91, 101, 111, 114, 36, 151, 153,
166, 169, 191, 194, 197, 198, 201, 205, 206,
210, 211, 217, 229, 232, 235, 237, 242, 243,
252, 253, 260, 266, 268, 270, 282, 340, 341,
342, 343
Abscesses, 37, 48, 52, 74, 111, 113, 115, 162
Acupuncture, 147, 148, 149
Alcohol, 34, 61,- 64, 66, 67, 84, 97, 105, 106, 134,
135, 155, 163, 165, 167, 171, 180, 182, 183,
207, 225, 236, 239, 240, 248, 250, 254, 258,
265, 275, 282, 292, 311, 355
Amebiasis, 95, 96
Aminosalicylates (5-ASA), 151, 152
Anastomosis, 143
Anemia, 53, 72, 86, 96, 97, 111, 159, 199, 219, 252,
258, 260, 269, 271, 280, 194, 302, 311
Angiosarcoma, 66, 68
Ankylosing spondylitis, 53, 74, 77, 78, 351
Antibiotics, 57, 59, 73, 75, 94, 96, 116, 120, 123,
124, 147, 151, 152, 157, 158, 166, 171, 172,
198, 205, 207, 212, 219, 251, 259, 261, 277, 335
Anticoagulants, 102, 103
Antidepressant medications, 130, 131, 132, 134, 135
Anus, 21, 33, 40, 42, 54, 56, 92, 110, 111, 144 - 146,
341
Appendicitis, 48, 197, 252, 340
Appendix, 31, 32, 48
Arthritis, 53, 71, 72, 74, 77, 78, 138, 139, 141, 155,
159, 191, 194, 203, 230, 231, 238, 257, 258,
259, 260, 269, 285

Arterial blood clots, 98
Atrial fibrillation, 100
Ascending Colon, 32

B

Back problems, 78
Bacteria, 31, 33, 34, 43, 44, 48, 57, 61, 75, 91, 92,
    94, 117, 118, 121, 149, 157, 158, 159, 161, 162,
    166, 192, 209, 233, 243, 251, 294, 326, 327,
    329, 330, 331 - 335
Barium x-ray, 108, 110
    Enema, 109, 110
    Oral, 108, 110
Bile, 22, 24, 26, 33, 34, 35, 48, 53, 58, 59, 61, 67,
    68, 70, 86, 87, 90, 170, 191, 195, 251, 328, 333,
    336
Bile duct, 24, 35, 53, 58, 59, 61, 67, 68, 86, 87, 90,
191, 195, 251
Blood clots, 97, 98, 99, 100 - 102, 120, 192, 220,
    230
    arterial, 98
    causes, 99
    diagnosing, 101
    prevention, 103
    symptoms, 100
    treatment, 102
    venous, 98
Bone thinning, see Osteoporosis, 81
Bones, 10, 81, 82, 83, 84, 174, 243
    types, 81
    understanding your, 82
    stopping calcium loss, 82
Bowel, 30, 36, 37, 38, 39, 40, 43, 44, 48, 49, 50 - 52,
    55, 56, 57, 58, 74, 77, 78, 85, 86, 92, 93, 108,
    109, 110, 111, 116, 119, 120 - 123, 144 - 146,

C

365

Depression; see Clinical Depression
Descending colon, 32, 40
Diabetes, 71, 72, 149, 154, 186, 199, 208, 220, 221,
    230, 231, 240, 254, 255, 269, 284, 293
Diabetic gastroparesis, 107
Diagnosis, 108 - 112, 147, 339, 340
    Diarrhea, 36, 38, 42, 48, 53, 55, 59, 95, 101,
    111, 114, 122, 134, 136, 146, 147, 151, 153,
    162, 166, 170, 173, 174, 177, 179, 182, 183,
    190, 191, 192, 194, 196, 198, 201 - 208, 211,
    213, 216 - 218, 224, 226 - 228, 230, 232 - 235,
    237, 238, 242, 243, 251, 252, 257, 260, 263,
    265, 269, 270, 272 - 274, 278, 280, 282, 289,
    291 - 293, 295, 300, 301, 303, 307, 311, 313,
    320, 330, 336, 339, 340 - 344
Diet, 18, 43, 50, 54, 63, 82 - 85, 89, 90, 93, 97, 117,
    146, 149, 153, 170, 173, 174, 178, 179, 184,
    198, 238, 253, 281, 289, 295, 296, 339
Digestive System, 21, 22, 23, 24, 27, 28, 30, 31, 42,
    51, 53, 57, 119, 120, 121, 147, 251
    anatomy, 27
    process, 21
    regulators, 22
    nerves, 23
    juices, 24
Digital rectal exam, 111
Disease maintenance, 173
DNA abnormalities, 44, 327
Doppler ultrasound, 101
Dorsal Sacroiliac Ligament, 79
Drug treatment, 137
Duodenum, 30, 105
Dysplasia, 40, 54

E
Embolism, see Pulmonary Embolism

Embolus, 98
Emotional impact of IBD, see Children, emotional
    impact
Emotional stress, 149, 176
Endoscopic Retrograde
    Cholangiopancreatopraphy, 58, 68
Endoscopy, 108
Enemas, 109, 110, 153, 161, 163, 175
Enteral nutritional, 120
Enzymes, 22, 23, 24, 25, 26, 27, 30, 31, 35, 90, 102,
    122, 297, 299, 326
    brush border, 31
    pancreatic, 22, 23, 25, 26, 35, 90
    protein digestion, 23
Epidemiology, 41
Erosive esophagitis, 107, 270
Erythema nodosum, 53, 72, 73, 74
Esophagus, 23, 25, 28, 62, 104, 105, 192, 220, 236,
269
Exercise, 46, 50, 55, 77, 78, 84, 85, 100, 103, 143,
    155, 174, 242, 253, 328
Eye inflammation, 78

F
Families' effect, 44, 45, 176
Family history, 72, 100
Fats, 22, 26, 170, 180, 254, 297
Feces, 33, 52, 144, 145, 270
Females and males (CD), 17
Fertility, 113, 114, 124, 152, 252
Fever, 38, 39, 42, 48, 52, 53, 56, 58, 59, 54, 68, 73,
    95, 100, 111, 123, 151, 153, 156, 190, 199, 201,
    202, 203, 206, 211, 213, 217, 219, 223, 226,
    227, 230, 234, 238, 242, 243, 244, 245, 247,
    250, 257, 260, 262, 265, 267, 269, 270, 272,
    274, 278, 282, 305
                        367

I

Irritable Bowel Syndrome (IBD), 38, 85, 185

J

Joints, 53, 76, 77, 203, 212, 213, 220, 260
J-pouch, 145, 146, 147

K

Kidney stones, 87, 88, 89, 269, 283, 292
   passing stones, 87
   symptoms, 87, 88
Klatskin tumor, 68

L

Lactose intolerance, 26, 93, 173
Laparoscopy, 56
Large intestine, 30, 31, 32, 33, 36, 39, 42, 48, 123,
   164, 233, 289, 339
Laxatives, 63, 85, 86, 174, 175, 176, 210, 331, 332,
   333
Lithotripsy, 88
Liver, 21, 22, 24, 26, 27, 29, 30, 31, 33 - 35, 53, 55,
   57, 59, 60 - 72, 86, 96, 102, 134, 157, 159, 164,
   165, 166, 171, 181, 192, 195, 196, 200, 203,
   211, 215, 223, 225, 228, 233, 239, 243, 248,
   251, 254, 258, 260, 270, 271, 280, 281, 283,
   292, 297, 299, 305, 310, 311, 326, 330, 331, 333
   cancers of, 64 - 70
   cirrhosis, 61
   hepatitis, 59
Low-fat diets, 289
Lower GI, 109
Lumenal surface, 30

M

Magnetic resonance angiogram, 101
Magnetic resonance imaging (MRI), 68
370

372

Pyoderma gangrenosa, 53, 74, 75, 76
Psychotherapy, 149

R

Rectal exam; see Digital Rectal Exam
Rectum, 31, 32, 33, 36, 38, 40, 49, 54, 65, 92, 109,
    110, 143, 144, 145, 161, 210, 244
Recurrence after surgery, 137, 143, 162
Relapse, 17, 41, 42, 117, 118, 136, 156, 173, 176
Remission, 19, 42, 94, 114, 116, 136, 137, 151, 153,
    159 – 162, 165, 166, 169, 173, 285
Rugae, 29

S

Sacroiliac, 75 - 78
Sacrotuberous Ligament, 79, 80
Sacrosipinous Ligament, 80
Saliva, 24, 25, 28
Scarring, 48, 52, 55, 58, 62, 63, 74, 104, 113, 267
Selective Serotonin Reuptake Inhibitors (SSRI), 132
Short bowel syndrome, 122
Sigmoiditis, 36
Sigmoidoscopy, 39, 40, 109, 110
Skin Problems, 163
Skin tags in anus, 48
Skip areas, 36 – 38
Skeleton, 81
Small bowel, 30, 48, 55, 119, 145, 174, 275
Small bowel obstruction, 55
Smoking, 83, 84, 100, 103, 105, 137, 143, 236, 265
Spastic colon, 38
Sphincter muscles, 33
Stoma, 145
Stomach, 21 – 30, 56, 57, 62, 65, 92, 104 – 109, 160,
    161, 192, 195, 197, 198, 201 – 206, 208, 211,
    212, 215 – 217, 222, 223, 226, 230 - 234, 236,